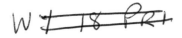

nking

ng for

dents

ORMATION SERVICE

WEAR VALLEYS

TION TRUST

PARK HOSPITAL

OUGH

Transforming Nursing Practice series

Transforming Nursing Practice is the first series of books designed to help students meet the requirements of the NMC Standards and Essential Skills Clusters for new degree programmes starting from 2011. Each book addresses a core topic, and together they cover the generic knowledge required for all fields of practice. Every book meets the main themes in the new standards by:

- building critical thinking, independent learning and decision-making skills;
- linking theory to practice;
- promoting partnership working with service users and other health and social care professionals;
- exploring the changing working environments nurses will face in the future.

Accessible and challenging, *Transforming Nursing Practice* helps nursing students prepare for the demands of future healthcare delivery.

Series editors:

Dr Shirley Bach, Head of the School of Nursing and Midwifery at the University of Brighton and Dr Mooi Standing, Principal Lecturer/Enterprise Quality Manager in the Department of Nursing and Applied Clinical Studies, Canterbury Christ Church University.

Titles in the series:

To order, contact our distributor: BEBC Distribution, Albion Close, Parkstone, Poole, BH12 3LL. Telephone: 0845 230 9000, email: **learningmatters@bebc.co.uk**. You can also find more information on each of these titles and our other learning resources at **www.learningmatters.co.uk**. Many of these titles are also available in various ebook formats. Please visit the website above for more information.

Critical Thinking and Writing for Nursing Students

Bob Price and Anne Harrington

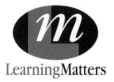

First published in 2010 by Learning Matters Ltd
Reprinted 2010 and 2011

British Library Cataloguing in Publication Data
A CIP record for this book is available from the British Library

ISBN: 978 1 84445 366 5

Adobe ebook   ISBN: 978 1 84445 689 5
EPub ebook   ISBN: 978 1 84445 688 8
Kindle   ISBN: 978 1 84445 985 8

Cover design by Toucan Design
Project management by Diana Chambers
Typeset by Kelly Winter
Printed and bound in Great Britain by TJ International Ltd, Padstow, Cornwall

Learning Matters Ltd
20 Cathedral Yard
Exeter EX1 1HB
Tel: 01392 215560
E-mail: info@learningmatters.co.uk
www.learningmatters.co.uk

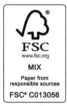

FSC
www.fsc.org
MIX
Paper from
responsible sources
FSC® C013056

Contents

Foreword

This invaluable book is a welcome and necessary addition to the *Transforming Nursing Practice* series, given the importance of developing and applying critical thinking and writing skills in nursing. Bob Price and Anne Harrington thoughtfully and imaginatively present critical thinking, reflecting and scholarly writing as essential nursing crafts which can be learned, practised and continually developed to succeed both in written assessments to register as a nurse, and for the lifelong learning necessary to maintain practice as a competent nurse. As such, the book will have particular appeal to pre-registration nursing students but it will also be of interest to qualified nurses on continuing professional development programmes.

Given the book's focus on enabling readers to write reflectively and critically, it is (perhaps more than any other book in the series) open to scrutiny regarding the presentation of material. The authors have risen to the challenge by successfully demonstrating the skills they describe and sincerely hope readers will emulate. They argue that good scholarly writing consists of completeness/coherence in structuring work; authority in presenting supportive and persuasive arguments; and clarity and precision which enables others to question and review their reasoning. In 'practising what they preach', the book is logically structured in three parts: 1) explaining concepts of critical thinking, reflecting, scholarly writing in an accessible, reader-friendly manner; 2) utilising experience of four nursing students to show how they progressed on a journey of self-discovery and enlightenment in their personal/professional development while negotiating lectures, workshops, clinical practice placements and computerised information technology settings; and 3) the inclusion of numerous, well-constructed activities inviting readers to question, explore and evaluate key concepts.

After reading and hopefully applying what can be learned from this book, readers will be very well equipped to understand how to reflect, analyse, critically review and articulate nursing experience and relevant theoretical or research perspectives. This includes making sense of formal learning opportunities such as lectures, workshops and computerised learning, as well as relatively informal learning opportunities with mentors during practice placements. The book is well referenced with up-to-date sources for further reading by more inquisitive readers, as well as useful websites. In addition, the authors have included helpful specimen analytical and reflective written assignments by students on the Learning Matters website. This is particularly useful for demonstrating how students negotiated and met the challenges of reflecting, analysing and articulating their nursing knowledge. The inclusion of theoretical/ analytical and experiential/reflective knowledge complements other existing or forthcoming books for nursing students by Learning Matters including *Understanding Research for Nursing*

Students, *Reflective Practice in Nursing*, *Evidence-Based Practice in Nursing*, and *Clinical Judgement and Decision Making for Nursing Students*. In keeping with other books in the series, this book clearly links contents to NMC standards for pre-registration nursing education.

Dr Mooi Standing
Series Editor

Acknowledgements

We would like to gratefully acknowledge the contributions of Stewart, Fatima, Raymet and Gina, who very generously agreed to explore critical thinking and reflection with us through their own work. Thanks go too to Gavin McNally and Ali Saher, students of City University, Community Health Sciences Department, and Sally Thorpe, Academic Adviser, School of Nursing and Midwifery at City University, who kindly read a number of the chapters.

Finally, all authors owe a debt of gratitude to families who patiently wait while books are written. Irrespective of what the book is about the wait is the same and the patience central to success. We are surrounded by supportive people. Thank you all.

About the authors

Bob Price is Director, Postgraduate Awards in Advancing Healthcare Practice at the Open University, an educational consultant, coach and an experienced writer of continuing professional development articles on thinking and learning with RCN Publishing journals. Bob has developed a number of courses on skills development, including those designed to assist students to analyse their own abilities and opportunities. A passionate educator, Bob has assisted students at every level from pre-registration programmes of study up to and including Doctor of Philosophy. Bob's doctoral thesis was on the negotiation of learning and strategies used by students and tutors to develop scholarly and professional forms of expression.

Anne Harrington is senior lecturer in law and ethics, management and education at City University. Anne has been teaching for nearly twenty years, and is passionate about supporting and enhancing students' learning experience. Her PhD in Education focused on the students' experience of academic support in higher education and reported that many of them who had their prior academic education overseas found it difficult to develop critical and analytical thinking when writing their essay.

Introduction

The ability to think critically, to reflect upon experience and then to write about such matters in a convincing fashion is central to your success on a programme of nursing studies. This book is designed to assist you with this process – the making sense of things that you read, hear, observe and experience, its translation into learning and representation within academic forms of writing set by the university. While other texts exist that describe reasoning and reflection, this one locks these skills into the process of learning and writing. However skilled you are as a critical thinker or as a reflector on practice, such abilities avail you little if you are then unable to express your learning to others.

Nursing presents us with a flood of information – gleaned from lectures, workshops, programmes of reading and what you discover during clinical placements. All of this has to be processed, and turned into that which you can use as a nurse. Processing this information in the right way takes time and benefits from wise counsel. You will naturally wish to liaise closely with your tutors as part of this work. As you sit down to think about what you have learned, though, and as you prepare essays and reflective journals, and revise for assessments, we believe that this textbook, ever present and available for consultation, will prove valuable.

Who is this book for?

We have written this book for a wide variety of students of nursing; certainly those who are completing their first course of studies leading to nurse registration, but those too who are continuing their studies thereafter and who perhaps have misgivings about their ability to write well. While we regularly refer to the UK's Nursing and Midwifery Council's *Standards for pre-registration nursing education* (NMC, 2010b), the book will, we believe, also serve well in other countries. Sound critical thinking and writing are of concern everywhere! Because the book starts from basics, it is designed to reassure and support those who may not have studied for some while. We begin with the assumption that critical thinking, reflecting and writing are three of the craft skills of nursing. Our approach here is based on our experience of designing and delivering open and flexible learning study materials, which might be worked through by a nurse planning for a course as well as those who are already enrolled.

Much of what is best in nursing is defined by the way in which we deliver care as much as what is provided. The way we listen, explore anxieties and needs, or suggest solutions demonstrates what is skilful about nursing. For this reason, reading this textbook will start you on a journey where you discover how best to use your experience in the service of others. This is a process that draws heavily upon making sense of practice, exploring what you believe is best within nursing care and planning future development that assists you to express your thinking more effectively.

Critical thinking and reflecting

One of the earliest discoveries made by nurses during their courses of study is how often the word 'critical' appears in their work. In the clinical context the word carries connotation of risk and the need for urgent intervention: a patient is critically ill, the next stage of treatment is critical. It can sometimes suggest that deterioration has set in or that we have not acted as proactively as we might. Used in this sense, the nurse quickly realises the need for precision and judgement, the requirement to do the right thing, in the right way and at the right time. In the academic context, critical takes on several different meanings. You are asked to 'critically discuss', to 'critically evaluate', to 'critically explore' a subject, and here it slowly becomes apparent that to be critical involves different things dependent on the teaching or assessment involved. For example, to be critical in this context might mean to discriminate between what is right and wrong, defensible and indefensible. However, it might also involve making judgements about what is influential here. Unfortunately, not all nursing course assessments spell out the sense in which the term critical is being used, so it is sometimes necessary to check with your tutor what the assessment requirements are.

In this textbook we use the term 'critical thinking' in a precise way. It describes the process by which we develop powers of analysis and investigation, and enhance our ability to discriminate what is relevant and to discern what might prove most helpful. Critical thinking involves judgement and nurses are frequently assessed with regard to their ability to judge and demonstrate skills and make appropriate decisions (Thompson and Dowding, 2009). A competent nurse is one who selects the relevant information to plan a course of action and then judges what is best to do in a given circumstance. The nurse has to be competent in managing risk. As well as this, though, the nurse needs to carry on learning and to grow professionally through experience. We are best placed to improve care where we have the capacity to reason what is not yet understood and what will enable us to be more imaginative, sensitive, respectful or efficient and effective in what we do.

While 'critical' is sometimes encountered in a more destructive form within practice (e.g., where practitioners belittle others' shortfalls), this is not the sense in which we will use it here. Indeed, we venture the view that the individual who criticises without consideration of what is learned through the experience isn't demonstrating either scholarship or professionalism.

It is likely that you have already engaged in reflection as part of previous studies and while growing up. For example, at school you perhaps judged which subjects to take to examination, based on your past comfort with them in class. However, in nursing reflection has a very important and specific role. Reflection is the process that assists nurses to make sense of the practice world around them, and to understand the risks, challenges and opportunities there (Howatson-Jones, 2010). Because nurses are asked to use their experience and their insights as part of nursing care, reflection takes on a special meaning. While at least some of your teaching in college starts with concepts or theories that describe the world of healthcare, much of what you learn through practice starts from episodes of care that are much more ambiguous. We have to make sense of what is going on and decide how best to proceed when at least some information is currently unavailable to us. The process of reflection then is central to nurses' learning and must be combined with theory in order to suggest how best to work next. It can tell us a great deal about our goals and values, beliefs and attitudes as well as what experience offers. Not surprisingly, then, both critical thinking and reflection are centre stage within this textbook. Critical thinking engages our reasoning as we ponder theories, arguments and debates, while reflection does the same as we contemplate experience.

How this book is set out

This text is set out in three parts. You will certainly benefit from reading it cover to cover, but it will also serve you when you wish to 'dip into' particular chapters later. Part 1 of the book consists of three chapters that introduce you in an accessible way to the three important concepts that feature in this book: critical thinking, reflecting and scholarly writing. Securing a basic idea about what these concepts are all about will help you make a great deal more sense of what is asked of you within the nursing syllabus.

Part 2 of the textbook concerns the use of reasoning and reflection within different contexts. We help you to understand what is involved in getting the most from lectures, workshops and clinical placements, and while using electronic media in your learning. While it may seem obvious that we listen when attending a lecture, for instance, we suggest in Chapter 4 that you can gain much more if you understand the process of lecturing and how this is used by tutors to further your education. Studying the chapters in Part 2 of this book will help you to become a more effective gatherer and processor of nursing information.

If Part 2 is about the process of learning, then Part 3 is about the process of expressing what you have learned. We assist you with the matter of writing different sorts of essays (analytical and reflective), and with building a portfolio that helps you to demonstrate progress and plan future learning.

Learning features

Throughout the book, you will find activities that will help you to make sense of, and learn about, the material being presented by the authors.

Some activities ask you to reflect on aspects of practice, or your experience of it, or the people or situations you encounter. *Reflection* is an essential skill in nursing, and one that helps you to understand the world around you and often to identify how things might be improved. Other activities will help you develop key skills, such as your ability to *think critically* about a topic in order to challenge received wisdom, or your ability to *research a topic and find appropriate information and evidence*, and to be able to *make decisions* using that evidence in situations that are often difficult and time-pressured. Finally, communication and working as part of a team are core to all nursing practice, and some activities will ask you to carry out *group activities* or think about your *communication skills* to help develop these.

All the activities require you to take a break from reading the text, think through the issues presented and carry out some independent study, possibly using the internet. Where appropriate, there are sample answers presented at the end of each chapter, and these will help you understand more fully your own reflections and independent study. Remember, academic study will always require independent work; attending lectures will never be enough to be successful on your programme, and these activities will help to deepen your knowledge and understanding of the issues under scrutiny and give you practice at working on your own.

You might want to think about completing these activities as part of your personal development plan (PDP) or portfolio. After completing the activity, write it up in your PDP or portfolio in a section devoted to that particular skill, then look back over time to see how far you are developing. You can also do more of the activities for a key skill in which you have identified a weakness, as this will help to build your skill and confidence in this area.

Because we know that case study illustrations of scholarly writing can prove very helpful indeed, we have positioned two examples of essays (one analytical and one reflective) on the publisher's website (**www.learningmatters.co.uk/nursing**). Each of these is free to download and for you to use as you think further about essay writing. While it is natural to feel anxious, perhaps even apprehensive about your studies, working with this book and its case studies should significantly improve your chances of not only doing well on your course, but enjoying study as well!

Nursing and Midwifery Council competencies

For those readers who are studying nursing courses within the UK, the NMC has established *Standards for Pre-registration Nursing Education*, which are standards of competence to be met by applicants to different parts of the register, and which it considers necessary for safe and effective practice. In addition to the competencies, the NMC has set out specific skills that nursing students must be able to perform at various points of an education programme. These are known as *Essential Skills Clusters* (ESCs). Critical thinking, reflection and writing have widespread relevance across all nursing competencies and ESCs. Therefore, we have, at the start of each chapter, identified those to which we think our material relates very closely, and which assist the reader to achieve the requirements for registration as a nurse.

This book includes the latest standards for 2010 onwards, taken from *Standards for Pre-registration Nursing Education* (NMC, 2010b). For links to the pre-2010 standards, please visit the website for the book at **www.learningmatters.co.uk/nursing**.

Part 1

Understanding thinking, reflecting and writing

Chapter 1

Critical thinking

NMC Standards for Pre-registration Nursing Education (2010)

This chapter will address the following competencies.

Domain: Professional values

8. All nurses must practise independently, recognising the limits of their competence and knowledge. They must reflect on these limits and seek advice from, or refer to, other professionals where necessary.
9. All nurses must appreciate the value of evidence in practice, be able to understand and appraise research, apply relevant theory and research findings to their work, and identify areas for further investigation.

(The ability to think critically and to distinguish what constitutes critical thought is key to appreciating the extent of current knowledge, that derived from different sources and that which might be used for different purposes.)

Domain: Nursing practice and decision making

Generic standard for competence: . . . Decision-making must be shared with service users, carers and families and **informed by critical analysis** of a full range of possible interventions . . .

1. All nurses must use up-to-date knowledge and evidence to assess, plan, deliver and evaluate care, communicate findings, influence change and promote health and best practice. They must make person-centred, evidence-based judgments and decisions, in partnership with others involved in the care process, to ensure high quality care. They must be able to recognise when the complexity of clinical decisions requires specialist knowledge and expertise, and consult or refer accordingly.

Domain: Leadership, management and team working

4. All nurses must be self-aware and recognise how their own values, principles and assumptions may affect their practice. They must maintain their own personal and professional development, learning from experience, through supervision, feedback, reflection and evaluation.

By the end of this chapter you will be able to:

- define critical thinking in your own practical terms using illustrations as necessary;
- with reference to different components of critical thinking, discuss why this skill is so important in nursing;
- summarise different aptitudes associated with critical thinking;
- indicate your level of confidence associated with each of the aptitudes of critical thinking, noting those that you hope to develop further in the future;
- describe what constitutes more sophisticated forms of critical thinking.

Introduction

Decision making, leadership and ethical practice are all founded upon an ability to think critically. We use critical thought to select resources, to utilise knowledge and to evaluate evidence. We have all been involved in reasoning throughout our lives, but it is highly likely that a lot of that has been conducted without a great deal of scrutiny. Many of the past decisions that we have made have been managed in a tacit way, that is, without great analysis. To be successful nurses, though, we need to practise the skill of critical thinking in a more conscious way. Not only do we need to discover what we have learned, but we need to understand how we have learned it. In this way we equip ourselves with the means to go on learning, even when our formal education is complete.

In this chapter we first explore why critical thinking is important in nursing, before unpicking what critical thinking typically consists of. The first of these is important as it explains why it is worth putting so much effort into the development of this skill. The second is relevant because, unless we can describe the component parts of critical thinking, it is difficult to practise the skill with any conviction. The chapter ends with some suggestions on how you can enhance your critical thinking.

To help you explore this subject matter we are going to introduce you to four student nurses. We will be returning to Stewart, Fatima, Raymet and Gina periodically throughout the book, but the discussions in this chapter focus on some of their early course learning.

Defining critical thinking

Before we turn to these matters, let us start by offering a first definition of what we mean by critical thinking. As Moon (2008) notes, a definition is difficult to pin down and each represents something of a compromise. However, it seems important to share with you our opening premises. Critical thinking for us is:

A process, where different information is gathered, sifted, synthesised and evaluated, in order to understand a subject or issue. Critical thinking engages our intellect (the ability to discriminate, challenge and argue), but it might engage our emotions too. To think critically we need to take account of values, beliefs and attitudes that shape our perceptions. Critical thinking then is that which enables the nurse to function as a knowledgeable doer – someone who selects, combines, judges and uses information in order to proceed in a professional manner.

                                                        Critical thinking

As you continue with your reading and revisit critical thinking in clinical placement, consider our definition and decide whether there is anything that you might add to or adjust concerning it. You may discover, for instance, that critical thinking is strongly affected by context. For example, where risk is a key consideration, there may be a much greater emphasis on making sound judgements.

As this activity is based on your own reflection, there is no answer at the end of the chapter.

Why critical thinking is important

Four student nurses have met up over coffee to discuss some of the challenges of completing a nursing studies course. While their studies are interesting, they all acknowledge that learning can be difficult because of the critical thinking required.

Activity 1.2   *Reflection*

Look now at the accounts in the box below of critical thinking challenges reported by these four students.

- Have you encountered similar concerns?
- Why do you think that making connections between teaching and practice (Stewart), managing uncertainty(Fatima), dealing with large volumes of information (Raymet), and knowing how, as well as what, to do (Gina) tells us about the importance of critical thinking in nursing?

We offer our own brief answers at the end of this chapter.

Case study: Four accounts of critical thinking challenges

Stewart: 'Have you noticed how hard it can be to connect up the stuff we are taught about pharmacology or physiology with what we see during our time on the ward? I feel so slow, sorting out what from that teaching I need to apply in the clinical setting!'

Fatima: 'For me it's the uncertainty. I long for a right answer, something that I know is sure, correct and a lot of what we're learning about . . . for instance ethics, isn't so clear cut.'

Raymet: 'I agree! But have you noticed just how much information there is? t's like they fill up your kit bag with everything you could ever want and then leave you to decide when to pull it out. The sheer volume is worrying.'

Gina: 'I wouldn't disagree with any of those points. But have you noticed how important it is to understand processes as well as purposes? You quickly know what you should do, but how to do it is something more complex. It's that which I find myself admiring nurses for. They can do things that I haven't begun to tackle.'

You may already be empathising with these four students, each of whom captures something about critical thinking in nursing. Nursing practice relies heavily on the skills of the nurse and central among these is the ability to reason. Gobet (2005) explains that all skills are made up of a series of component parts and that it is the way in which these are combined and used that determines how skilful the practice seems (see Figure 1.1). Nurses develop templates in their own minds to determine how best to work, but practice constantly demands that we adjust these ideas, combining and recombining the different skill components in ways to suit prevailing conditions.

In the case study that we just looked at, Stewart refers to the first of these components. While his first concerns are about the application of theory, this only becomes important because, without clear guidance on this, Stewart is unsure how best to proceed. If we are going to deliver good nursing care we have to know how to combine and apply information. We have to be able to declare certain things (as true, sound, proven, relevant) if we are to develop the confidence to proceed. Critical thinking in this context therefore involves the piecing together of bits of information from several different sources, in ways that help us to determine what is happening. A very simple example makes the point. When Stewart cares for a patient receiving drugs to lower blood pressure, Stewart would need to know something about the action of the chosen medication (theory), its effect on the physiology of the body (research evidence) and how this presented in terms of base-line observations (experience), in order to make sense of what he then witnessed. He could only declare what was normal, expected or

Figure 1.1: Components of nursing skill.

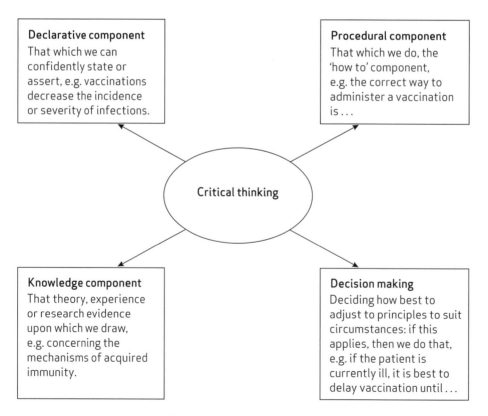

Source: After the work of Gobet (2005).

problematic if he was able to combine and evaluate information in this way. Stewart proceeds on the basis of what he is confident that he understands and can promote or recommend as beneficial to others.

Fatima refers to a second important component of critical thinking, *decision making*. There is often no 'one size fits all' solution. Fatima is keenly aware that the nurse has to deal with uncertainty, sometimes waiting to gather more information before making a decision. Living with such uncertainty, especially in clinical practice, is what can seem stressful for nurses. They have to learn to read developing situations and to weigh the merits of different courses of action. The process of reasoning, therefore, is important to nursing because it provides a discipline for deciding how best to proceed in practice. If we simply react instinctively, and if we do as we have always done because it worked with other patients, the nurse might make a mistake.

What Raymet is discussing concerns *knowledge*. Professional practice is under-pinned by a raft of knowledge and this comes from many sources: research, experience, theory and work in related fields (e.g., counselling or medicine). We can only reason effectively if we have amassed a sufficient quantity of high-quality knowledge. Reasoning then involves several things, accepting some sorts of knowledge as important, but standing ready to challenge others. As well as choosing what knowledge to use in practice, the nurse needs to know when to discard knowledge and search for something more robust. So, while Stewart is concerned with what information fits a particular situation (application), Raymet is concerned with judging the worth of information (currency and validity). Is it adequate, coherent and sufficient? As part of your course studies you will be introduced to ways of critiquing research evidence, but that same quizzical attitude towards knowledge remains important in other areas as well, for example where competing claims are made with regard to the proper or priority work of the nurse.

Lastly, Gina refers to the *process* part of the skill. Reasoning is concerned not only with deciding what knowledge is appropriate, determining what is true, safe or effective and making judicious decisions, it is concerned with how you order your work. When a nurse gives an injection he or she combines different sorts of knowledge to a clear purpose, but also determines the right order in which to proceed. For example, the nurse forewarns the patient about the planned injection, secures consent and then ensures a private environment to help protect the patient's dignity. Knowing how to sequence work, how to refer, confer or consult, and how to secure important resources or feedback are process elements of reasoning as used in clinical practice.

It seems hardly surprising, then, that learning to nurse requires a lot of work and an appreciation of the ways in which nurses combine different things to work skilfully. No matter what part of your course you study, you will be engaged in critical thinking, combining and recombining the different components of nursing skill in order to proceed in ways that seem professional. Nursing practice has to be reasoned and the actions of the nurse reasonable. Indeed, in a court of law, judgments about whether a nurse's actions are negligent are based upon what a reasonable practitioner would do (Mardell and Serfozo, 2010). What Stewart and the others learn through their course is designed to enable them to work more safely, strategically, effectively (achieving required outcomes) and efficiently (using resources wisely).

Does the above information help explain why learning can make you feel both anxious and excited as you combine:

- ideas about what can be declared;
- underpinning knowledge;
- insights into how to proceed;
- with ways of making decisions?

Discuss with your colleagues which of the components seem most challenging to you. If you have these in common with others, consider whether they are something that you might discuss within a personal tutor group.

As this activity is based on your own reflection, there is no answer at the end of the chapter.

Making critical thinking work for you

Having identified the different components of critical thinking only helps you so far. You need to consider how you might actually use them to best effect and here aptitude, ability and readiness to proceed come into play. For example, if a nurse fails to ask questions (an aptitude) and accepts the status quo, few improvements in practice can be expected. Doing the same thing, in the same way, is unlikely to produce change.

Let's return again to the four nurses. In Table 1.1 the colleagues each suggest an aptitude that they think is important to the successful nurse.

Activity 1.4 *Critical thinking*

Study Table 1.1 and decide how important you rate the aptitude suggested by each of the student nurses (of great importance, of some importance, neither important nor unimportant, of little importance, of no importance).Write down a short rationale for each of your decisions. Are there any circumstances where the importance of an aptitude could change?

We supply brief answers of our own at the end of the chapter.

All of the aptitudes within this table have a justifiable role in critical thinking. It is significant that we think of these as aptitudes. This is because we have seen that students are either more or less inclined to engage in these, and more or less confident regarding them. Some people argue better than others; they are persuasive and able to convey their thinking clearly. Others are more imaginative and comfortable speculating about how nursing care could be. They speculate in safe places, away from the bedside, and discuss ideas with patients that sometimes transform the way in which care is delivered.

Table 1.1: Critical thinking aptitudes.

The student	The aptitude	Points made
Stewart	Asking questions	'If nurses don't ask questions about their work, they will never know what they don't know.'
Fatima	Discriminating	'Perhaps! But when you do know things you still have to decide what is relevant. We can't use every bit of information, we have to accept some information as being better for this situation.'
Raymet	Making arguments	'I wouldn't dismiss your points but here's a better one. Once you've decided that something is relevant you have to make arguments. I don't mean silly arguments, but the sort that help you defend what you think is best.'
Gina	Interpreting and speculating	'All worthy stuff . . . but where is imagination in all this? The best nurse I ever saw was someone who kept imagining what could be different. She was always thinking about better solutions.'

Activity 1.5   *Reflection*

What are your critical thinking aptitudes? For example, do you think that you are reasonably good at asking questions in a constructive way? Do you think that you can formulate arguments – ones that seem to help others understand the problem?

Don't worry if you feel your aptitudes are underdeveloped at this stage; we will be working on these again later and much of your course will involve encouraging you to improve these in turn.

As this activity is based on your own reflection, there is no answer at the end of the chapter.

We shall now examine each aptitude in more depth.

Asking questions

Asking questions is certainly important, but individuals vary in their level of confidence. Perhaps you worry that asking questions suggests an uncomfortable level of ignorance or gaps in your knowledge? Asking questions, though, and especially when working with professional colleagues, is at the heart of healthcare. For example, questions are frequently used to clarify the best care options and at best these involve patients in decisions made. All members of the team offer questions – ones that are designed to examine alternative explanations of what has been learned and what might resolve a problem in the future. Sometimes the more naive question is the one that transforms the team's understanding of a clinical situation.

You may hear nurse mentors rehearsing questions aloud as an aide to planning or adjusting care. 'These are some questions that I would ask myself at this stage about educating patients,' they might say! What does the patient need to know and master? When are they in the right position to start learning? However, asking questions in this way is not to trap ourselves in the realms of doubt. It is instead to suggest that we don't jump to conclusions and that we keep our understanding of situations open until we have enough evidence to support our interpretation of events.

Discriminating

There comes a stage where we have to discriminate between what is relevant or important, or what is true and what is false. Discrimination involves weighing information and determining what enables us to make arguments, such that might be supported by others. One example of discrimination in action is where nurses search for empirical evidence to support a given practice. The nurses reason that the information supplied through research studies is superior to that derived from anecdote, at least where the design of research has been rigorous and clearly described.

Returning to the above example of a skilful mentor in action, we might imagine him or her next also weighing up the case made by researchers in an article that the mentor has read. The article describes a study of how patients with diabetes were taught to care for themselves. The mentor might debate the following:

- Is what the authors claim true? (Truth might not be universal, as something that is defensible in one circumstance is not always so in another. For example, patients from one culture may have different expectations of learning from those of another.)
- Are there any competing explanations for this? (The mentor notes that, while the research data could certainly explain what happened, other things could too. In our example, that could be about what motivates patients to learn about self care.)
- Is the information coherent and its origins appropriately explained? (Our mentor might reasonably expect all the details of how the research was conducted to be available, the better to judge whether claims made there are supportable. In this example, did the researchers establish clearly at the outset what patients already knew about diabetes mellitus?)

Making arguments

Arguments are formulated about a variety of things: what should be done next, what this literature suggests is valuable, what constitutes patient-centred care. Arguments are necessary, as they explain the premises that underpin our action and why we are working to the goals that we do. As we shall see in later chapters, arguments are central to successful analytical essays and your ability to convince others within these. Arguments need to be measured, calm and well considered. Those that simply appeal to emotion won't help the nurse to make a case.

Our example mentor might accept that the research report shared was indeed relevant to our chosen practice setting, and that the design of the study was rigorous. The researchers have shown all their 'workings out' along the way. However, our mentor might then argue that, because there has been a local policy change associated with where patients are best educated (within the community as opposed to hospital), we cannot simply adopt the recommendations for practice contained in that research study. We must make some important adjustments that reflect rehabilitation in the community.

Activity 1.6   *Critical thinking*

In no more than two or three sentences, write out an argument now – one that you think is appropriately scholarly. For example, you might write an argument about what demonstrates patient-centred care.

Then note down what is it about your argument that you think makes it sound.

When you have finished, turn to the end of the chapter to learn about the features of a scholarly argument.

Interpreting and speculating

We have left speculation until last, and consider it extremely important. Successful nursing relies in significant part on nurses 'thinking outside the box', daring to consider options or solutions that are unfamiliar. Creativity and imagination therefore form a valuable part of critical thinking and one that can help nurses improve the lot of patients. In the following, Gina talks about her clinical mentor:

> *It was like a military campaign. My mentor pulled all the information together about teaching the diabetic patients and quickly realised that, with the staff available, they couldn't do it in the old familiar way. That was when she suggested that they should teach patients in groups and organise the sessions so the patients helped one another out. As the patients assisted one another my mentor watched them and decided who understood the insulin treatment best.*

How can we reason better?

However appealing it seems to place the above aptitudes in a set sequence and to say that this is the best or right way to reason, we have to acknowledge that critical thinking is a little less formulaic than this. Nurses often start by asking questions, but they could also start by preparing arguments before testing these out against what they read or see. We call tentative arguments of this kind 'working hypotheses' – draft explanations of what we think is happening and what will happen next. Reasoning therefore seems to work in two ways and sometimes in parallel:

- **Deductively**: we test working hypotheses to see whether what we predict is in fact the case (an example of this is when a theory of health beliefs is used to predict where the nurse can have greatest effect, for example persuading the patient to give up cigarette smoking).
- **Inductively**: we continue gathering information in order to formulate theories and explanations of what is happening. In this approach we speculate as we go, using our ideas to suggest where we might look next for valuable information. (An example of this is where the nurse builds a working theory of how best to break

bad news to patients or relatives. He or she uses experience with other patients to identify what seems most supportive.)

Critical thinking is in many instances like working on a jigsaw puzzle. We attend to different parts of the problem or need, making progress in one area because this seems necessary now. Problem-based learning courses emphasise exactly this process (Price, 2003a). Students are presented with outline case studies and search for further information in order to plan care. The process of learning to make sense of ambiguous situations is at the centre of study and replicates the conditions that are met in practice.

Working on your aptitudes enables you to develop progressively more sophisticated approaches to critical thinking. Moon (2008) summarises these as part of her wide-ranging discussion on ways of thinking about knowledge. Instead of seeing situations in deceptively simplistic terms, the thinker learns to explore the complexity of healthcare situations. The more sophisticated our reasoning, the more flexible and comfortable we become as we consider each problem, challenge or need in turn. We become better at making sense of what is happening, identifying what could happen next and how we might then best proceed.

Activity 1.7   *Decision making*

Look now at the ways of reasoning described in Table 1.2 and decide which you think are the more sophisticated forms of reasoning and which are the least sophisticated. Decide for yourself if you employ one of these approaches more than others.

As this activity is based on your own reflection, there is no answer at the end of the chapter.

Debate continues about what represents more or less sophisticated forms of reasoning, and nursing demands different forms of reasoning at different times; but here we venture the following. The least sophisticated forms of reasoning are what Baxter-Magolda (1992) calls absolute. At this level the individual is unable to see issues in 'shades of grey' or to accept that a range of possible perspectives could be taken on a subject. The thinker looks for certainty and only feels secure when matters have been decisively concluded: 'this is right, that is wrong, this is what we believe, this is what we don't believe'. If you are prone to thinking in this way, you might note how often you ask the tutor to be expert, to define what is 'correct'. While an absolute might be expected with regard to some areas of work, for example the right drug to use in an emergency, it is not something that is possible or even desirable in many other situations (e.g., finding the right ways to demonstrate that we are listening). We need to be more flexible in our approach. Absolute thinking is a common way of reasoning, especially at the start of a university education.

We have placed silent absorption next, at least where the individual feels incapable of comprehending what the important issues are. The thinker waits, soaking up more and more information in the hope that reasoning will be assisted by the accumulation of knowledge. In practice, this doesn't always work out. More information doesn't always lead to clarity and there is a need to ask questions and discuss ideas if we are to develop confidence in our reasoning. We add a caveat here, though, and note that some students come from a background (e.g., the Far East) where it is considered polite and appropriate

Table 1.2: Ways of reasoning.

Reasoning approach	Description
Independent knowing*	So much knowledge is constructed by people. For example, a dental appointment is understood (as good or bad) with regard to our previous experiences of dental treatment. So we search experience to suggest clues on how to think about things and then take up our position on that subject.
Contextual knowing*	We rely strongly on contexts to determine what we focus upon – what we accept as important and valuable. For example, we might suggest that the circumstances of a family of a dying patient strongly influence how they cope with news that the illness is incurable.
Transitional knowing*	Reasoning involves living with doubts, about what is true, best, defensible or important. We learn to wait and see and accept that right now several explanations of the situation might be supportable.
Silent absorption**	The individual absorbs and appreciates a growing volume of information, contemplating the same without necessarily venturing an opinion. For example, a student attends a series of lectures on physiology, venturing no opinion on what is discussed there until all the important facts are to hand.
Absolute knowing*	We search for what is right or wrong, them or us, making clear distinctions – that which is fact and that which is not. We search for the definitive answer that properly supports care decisions.

Source: Based on the typologies of Baxter Magolda (1992)* and Belenky et al. (1986)**.

not to intervene with questions, allowing the teacher or expert practitioner to complete their presentation. Where that then leads to the thinker summarising their own thoughts – their own grasp of wisdom – the reasoning remains sophisticated and can be described as cultural in nature. Where, though, the learner continues to accrue knowledge but struggles with understanding, opportunities to improve have been missed.

We put forward that transitional thinking comes next, suggesting that the thinker is ready to live with the uncertainties of knowledge, but is ready too to question as opportunities present. You will need to reason in this way, accepting that, in some clinical contexts, and pro temp, not all can be understood about a situation. Insights emerge from what is experienced and discussed and, in the meantime, it is necessary to remain alert to what experience or a carefully selected question can assist you with. For example, this happens as we monitor a developing illness in a patient and determine how best to modify treatment, controlling body temperature or adjusting fluid balance.

Contextual thinking is even more sophisticated and suggests that the thinker understands that there are lots of different truths in the world and what works in one context doesn't work in another. This is not to suggest that you have no principles or standards and that 'anything goes' within nursing. Principles and safe practice are important, but there may well be different ways of doing things within those parameters. A good example of this working well is where nurses explore with patients the nature of dignity. What represents dignified care can vary widely and takes into account patient expectations, lifestyle and custom (Wicks, 2007).

Independent thinking is arguably the most sophisticated form of reasoning and one that helps you to become more innovative over time. At this level you allow others to adopt their own position, and to develop arguments in support of the same, while you build your own case about the subject in hand. You carefully search what there is to support your own position, stand ready to change it if others can persuade you, and treat all discussion in a thoughtful and enquiring way. An example of this might be where the nurse adopts a clear and defensible stance associated with extended role, exploring its benefits in healthcare, but also considering the extent to which this fits with the nurse's own philosophy of care and career aspirations (Joel, 2009).

As you review your answers to Activity 1.7 don't be alarmed if you felt that your own thinking was near the bottom of this hierarchy! Students at university frequently need to work from the bottom. Moving from more familiar ways of reasoning to those that involve greater uncertainty and challenge means that you have to move out of your comfort zone. Excellent tutors are adept at helping students to do this, respecting their anxieties, but always searching for better ways to help them explore nursing. This is one of the key reasons why your course is likely to involve different sorts of learning activity (e.g., lectures, discussion groups, demonstrations, role play). Each in some regard practises you in different forms of reasoning and promotes what you will need to demonstrate in order to be successful practitioners.

CHAPTER SUMMARY

It is time now to sum up what has been shared in this chapter. We have introduced you to basic ideas about critical thinking and explained that it is a process – one that involves the gathering, receiving and processing of information in order to understand the world around you. It is important in nursing for a number of reasons: those associated with safety, with creativity, with problem solving and the management of a great deal of uncertainty that often attends patients and their needs. The discussion of Gobet's (2005) work emphasises that nurses need to be able to declare what they believe to be true and trustworthy, as the basis for subsequent action. Equally important is a grasp of process – how care is delivered, and what treatment works and why. Reasoning in this sense guides the nurse in a series of daily activities that help the patients with their needs. Another component of reasoning that makes it important is decision making – deciding what to do next when nurses and colleagues have incomplete information. Finally, knowledge accumulation and application are important. Nurses have to combine a lot of theoretical knowledge and know when to apply it, and reasoning is central to this work.

For reasoning to work in practice, though, and for the component parts of this skill to work together, nurses must develop certain aptitudes. These include asking questions, making arguments, speculating and discriminating. It is highly likely that there remains considerable scope for you to develop these further during the course of your studies. Rest assured, it is quite natural for students to have anxieties about these and tutors understand this! Part 2 of this book returns to many of these matters afresh.

Finally, we briefly explored ways in which we might recognise more sophisticated forms of reasoning. Some areas of nursing work will require these, for instance with regard to professional ethics, innovation in practice or the development of care philosophies that show how we work best with patients. Studying this material should have helped you to decide where your own reasoning has progressed to so far and to identify when it is improving in the future. Completion of the chapter activities will have afforded you the opportunity to do several things, including the preparation of arguments and identification of what within your reasoning is already well developed.

Activities: brief outline answers and reflections

Activity 1.2: Reflection (page 9)

Critical thinking challenges	Importance in nursing
Connecting abstract concepts or theories in teaching to clinical practice (Stewart)	Theories, frameworks and other descriptions are shorthand ways of describing the world of nursing. They can help us to anticipate what is important, safe or timely in what we do. But because practice circumstances vary so much, we have to be able to select and interpret what is most applicable from our teaching in practice. If we don't do that we are left frustrated that practice is not more like theory, or conversely that theory does not capture the reality of practice.
Managing uncertainty, making the best decision (Fatima)	Nurses rarely have the benefit of complete information as they deliver care, so sometimes we have to proceed on the basis of probabilities – deciding what seems best and what will be efficacious. We have to use judgement about information received and what this suggests it is important to do next.
Managing a volume of information (Raymet)	Just as sometimes we have too little information to plan care with, so sometimes we can have too much. It becomes difficult to decide what is most relevant. We therefore need to be able to discriminate what is important now.
Knowing what is important but also how to proceed (Gina)	Knowing how to care is important because nurses have to combine knowledge and skills – to combine facts with actions. It is this that makes care seem timely, sensitive, expert and insightful.

Activity 1.4: Critical thinking (page 12)

It may not surprise you to learn that we consider all the aptitudes discussed here to be important, but that judging when and where to use these is also necessary. For example, asking questions in a university discussion is likely to be welcomed, especially where you develop the ability to debate issues with study group peers and your tutor. However, asking questions should be handled rather differently in the clinical setting, as this is a place of 'public performance'. The questions that you pose to a senior nurse or doctor might, to a patient or relative, seem a direct challenge to their authority. Discussing each of these aptitudes in academic and clinical context use with your tutor should help you to make more successful transitions between campus and clinical placement.

Activity 1.6: Critical thinking (page 15)

Here is our example of an argument:

> *Patients who have recently suffered a major burn deal with physical deformity later than we might expect and this for three reasons. First, other physiological needs push to the fore, for example managing pain. In a series of 14 cases reviewed in our practice, concerns about safety and discomfort took precedence in the patients' minds. Second, patients suffer from information overload, as they have so many other things to deal with such as dressings and physiotherapy. We have catalogued over 50 pieces of information that we routinely ask burns patients to grapple with. Third, staff conspire to protect patients from distressing revelations. In our experience, mirrors are often removed from burns unit walls.*

In an argument an assertion is made. In this case, it is the point that patients deal with the distress of deformity rather later than other things. Support information is then added. This nurse uses evidence from practice. An argument therefore consists of an assertion and supports. In a subsequent argument you might consider the alternative case, where patients report early distress with their appearance. In this way you demonstrate the ability to weigh arguments before adopting a final position of your own.

Knowledge review

Having worked through this chapter, rate your understanding of the following topics as one of the following: poor, adequate, improving or excellent.

1. The different component parts of critical thinking (declarative, procedural, decision making, knowledge).
2. The different aptitudes needed to reason well (e.g., asking questions).
3. What is required if we are to think in a more sophisticated as well as a critical way.

Next, make a note of your personal progress as regards the different component parts of critical thinking, the different aptitudes and your level of reasoning (sophisticated or otherwise). Don't worry, the purpose of such notes is not to judge you; these simply form a starting point from which you proceed and that you can revisit after you have completed your reading of this book.

Further reading

Moon, J (2008) *Critical Thinking: An exploration of theory and practice.* London: Routledge.

This is a demanding but very valuable book about critical thinking and one that shows Moon's command of the literature. It is a book that is especially valuable for tutors. Moon catalogues why critical thinking is hard to describe and in Chapter 6 discusses 'academic assertiveness', something that is encouraged among nurse learners.

Jones, S (2009) *Critical Learning for Social Work Students*. Exeter: Learning Matters. Don't be put off by the title of this book, as many of the chapters within this readable book should be of interest to nurses as well. In Chapter 1, Sue Jones focuses heavily on the development of critical questions, one of the components of reasoning discussed here.

Useful websites

http://assets.cambridge.org/052100/9847/sample/0521009847ws.pdf
Alec Fisher (2001) What is critical thinking and how to improve it, Chapter 1 from *Critical Thinking: An introduction*. Cambridge: Cambridge University Press.
This free download of an excerpt chapter from a textbook on critical thinking provides supplementary information on the nature of assumptions and the questioning attitude needed to explore what we encounter. The author writes for a wide audience, but the ideas shared here are readily translated into the healthcare context and the chapter provides a very useful supplement for those who wish to explore the nature of critical thinking a little further.

www.criticalthinking.org/research/index.cfm (The Critical Thinking Community)
Critical thinking is widely taught as an academic subject in North America and this California-based site provides a number of resources for both those who teach it and those who try to develop critical thinking skills in association with the school or college course. The site offers a number of free downloads that explore the nature and teaching of critical thinking and will be of interest to all who are interested in developing critical thinking techniques.

www.humboldt.edu/~act/HTML/index.html (Argumentation and critical thinking tutorial, Humboldt State University)
Formal logic, the development of sound arguments and the scrutiny of arguments presented by others are excellent ways to exercise critical thought, both within educational courses and beyond. This site offers a series of interactive and informal tests that assist the visitor to check their powers of reasoning and to venture arguments that are logically sound.

Chapter 2

Reflecting

NMC Standards for Pre-registration Nursing Education (2010)

This chapter will address the following competencies.

Domain: Professional values

2. All nurses must practise in a holistic, non-judgmental, caring and sensitive manner that avoids assumptions; supports social inclusion; recognises and respects individual choice; and acknowledges diversity. Where necessary, they must challenge inequality, discrimination and exclusion from access to care.

Domain: Communication and interpersonal skills

1. All nurses must build partnerships and therapeutic relationships through safe, effective and non-discriminatory communication. They must take account of individual differences, capabilities and needs.

Domain: Leadership, management and team working

4. All nurses must be self-aware and recognise how their own values, principles and assumptions may affect their practice. They must maintain their own personal and professional development, learning from experience, through supervision, feedback, reflection and evaluation.

Chapter aims

By the end of this chapter you will be able to:

*   define reflection, indicating how a stated purpose can help to make reflections more critical;
*   distinguish the differences between reflecting in practice and on practice, detailing why they are different from one another;
*   identify six reasons why reflection is important in nursing, noting those that appear in most frequent use;

- discuss the best principles of reflection, identifying how you will proceed in the future;
- explain why it is important to ascertain course expectations associated with frameworks for reflection, and whether reflection should be practised at both the intimate and the skill review level.

Introduction

Nursing courses are strongly associated with the skill of reflection and for very good reasons as we shall see below. However, it is a skill that we have all engaged in and which we all use on a regular basis. It is one that is facilitated by the soap operas or reality shows that we see on television. What delights us here is the opportunity to debate what was said and done, and what might have been said or done as an alternative. Behaviour was 'wise', 'foolish', 'typical of that character' or 'critical to what happened next'. We are all armchair experts! Reflection is certainly a skill that we practise during or after important social encounters, for example a first meeting, a romantic date or a job interview.

In this chapter we start first with some distinctions between reflecting on the here and now and on what has gone before. This is an excellent way to focus our attention on reflection, because we believe that you will quickly note some practical differences between the two, and that this will help you discover just how important reflection can be. Next, we share our own definition of reflection and help you to identify why it is distinct from other forms of critical thinking. Reflection focuses on experience and admits feelings into the equation. We proceed then to a review of why reflection is so essential in nursing and why it is emphasised within your nursing course. While we as nurses are not the only healthcare professionals to reflect, we suspect that we use the skill more than many to explore our own roles and what nursing as a whole stands for and delivers. Finally, the chapter explores some of the best principles of reflection – things that you will need to take into account as you reflect alongside your course studies.

Let us begin by making a key distinction regarding the skill of reflection in action. It seems to us a fundamental one and something that helps to explain how reflection is used within the nursing course.

Activity 2.1   *Reflection*

Consider this suggestion: 'Reflection changes when we practise it after the event rather than during it.'

- Do you support this statement and if so why?
- What is qualitatively different about reflecting in practice rather than retrospectively on practice?

As this activity is based on your own reflection, there is no answer at the end of the chapter.

Schon (1987) certainly believes that reflecting on action is different from reflecting in action. If we reflect on the event as it unfolds, we have none of the benefits of calm introspection and time to consider at leisure the different options available to us. Against that, if we reflect long after the event, it is likely that memory may play tricks on us and we remember certain features of the event better than others. Have you noticed how, in childhood memory, snow at Christmas seemed more common? Reflecting in practice involves 'thinking on our feet'. We have to attend very quickly to what others say or do and accommodate the feelings that quickly well up inside us as we deal with the events as they unfold. We cannot pause the action in order to produce the sage-like response that we would love to deliver. Reflecting in action is in some sense rather 'raw', but perhaps all the more vivid for that. We can illustrate that with two short excerpts of reflection from an experienced staff nurse called Lauren. In the first extract Lauren is reflecting in action and in the second she reflects on action. It is important to note that in action reflections are usually unspoken. Speaking aloud our thoughts could prove problematic in many clinical settings!

Case study: Reflection in action and Reflecting on practice

Reflecting in action

Is this man going to hit me . . . he seems really angry? What does he want? I need to say something, do something that shows him that I respect his concerns. I need to suggest something. I know, I'll suggest that we talk in the relatives' room, but leaving the door open in case I need assistance. That shows I will give him time to tell me what worries him, and I'll remain safe! Yes, that seems to have worked, he is agreeing to accompany me. But he's still talking as we go – he's like a pressure cooker and I'm worried about how that will seem to the other relatives on the ward . . .

Reflecting on practice

The relative had suffered a major shock. He thought that he had nearly a week to prepare for his wife to come home and here she was ready to be discharged that afternoon! No wonder he was fuming. We were meeting our needs to make a bed available for someone else and foisting the patient back into his care at short notice. Colleagues could see that his wife required some more rehabilitation at home, so this was going to be a significant responsibility for him.

The above excerpts show just how different reflecting seems at these points. Notice the staccato way in which thoughts emerge when reflecting in action. There is a frantic search for meaning. Lauren has to work with her perceptions of what the relative is feeling as well as her own experiences of a confrontation. The reflections on action are evaluative and confident. Lauren can assert a great deal more about the origins of the problem.

In your course the opportunities to reflect on action may be legion. You will be asked to write reflective essays, and to develop case studies that explore the quality of care delivered to one or more patients. The very nature of recording reflections in a written account makes them retrospective in nature (we think faster than we can write). Opportunities to reflect in action and with support are much rarer. If you are fortunate, they occur with an experienced practical skills teacher or clinical mentor, who helps you to rehearse aloud your thinking within a psychologically safe environment (one where a reflective account doesn't alarm patients) (Price, 2005).

Defining reflection

The above early distinction between reflecting in practice and on practice serves us well, as we explore next the definition of reflection used within this book. Reflection is a skill used in two contexts – during events and after them. We think of reflection as a subset skill of critical thinking and one that is used in close association with experience. It involves the use of decision making (reflecting in action) and evaluation (reflecting on action). In both cases we are making sense of events around us and trying to use our personal aptitudes in order to work in ways that seem more sensitive and successful. For example, to reflect in action it is important that we are able to think of our own actions as we might when watching an actor on stage. We have to consider not only what happened and how we felt, but also what our own motives or goals might have been for that situation (Howatson-Jones, 2010).

To take the case of Lauren, there is a need to speculate about how we can best assist this angry relative to express his concerns, in a way that limits the risk of violence. This aptitude is called metacognition (Dunlosky and Metcalfe, 2008). It is the process of considering our own motives and actions as they work in concert with those of others involved in an event. Another important aptitude associated with reflection (especially on action) is empathy. We need to be able to appreciate the actions of others in context and with reference to circumstances that brought the event about (Slote, 2007).

We argue, then, that reflection is:

a process whereby experience is examined in ways that give meaning to interaction. We might examine the experience in real time or in retrospect. Because experience engages the emotions as well as reasoning, reflection needs to take account of the feelings engendered within an interaction and to allow that perceptions (how we interpret matters) may sometimes prove erroneous. While reflection is most closely associated with human interactions and especially clinical events, it is not limited to these. We may, for instance, reflect upon the written accounts of experiences, such as those shared by dying patients. Reflection may be used in the service of different nursing goals – those that are designed to tell us something about how we think, what we value and with regard to ways in which practice could be improved.

Activity 2.2   *Critical thinking*

Study the above definition now and make brief notes on why you think we have emphasised perception so strongly there. A hint that might help you comes from all those arguments that you may have shared regarding events in a reality TV show! Did you all agree on what happened and who was to blame for an unfortunate event? Notice, too, the point about reflection serving different purposes – those associated with personal insight and practice improvement. Why do you think it is important that we understand the motives for reflection?

We share brief responses to this activity at the end of the chapter.

Why reflecting is important

In Figure 2.1 we represent some of the reasons why reflection is so important in nursing. Just how apparent these are depends in part on how far you have progressed through your course of studies. Some of the rationale for reflection only really becomes apparent as you study within different learning environments and deal with different subjects within the curriculum.

Figure 2.1: Why reflection is important in nursing.

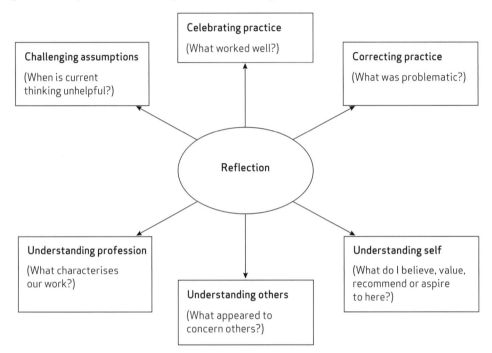

Activity 2.3   *Critical thinking*

Annotate Figure 2.1 with a score in each box to indicate how frequently you have observed reflection being used to that purpose in your course so far. So, for example, if it is used very frequently indeed, score it 3, if it used regularly score it 2, if it is used only occasionally score it 1, and if you have never seen it used for that purpose score it 0. If you date these scores, you can return to this activity later to see whether these have changed as your course progresses and your experience grows. Consider next whether reflection is primarily seen as a corrective tool or one that liberates nursing.

As this is a personal observation activity we don't provide answers of our own, but read on now to explore further the purposes of reflection in nursing.

Celebrating practice

Reflection on action can be put to excellent use to celebrate that practice which is successful and which exceeds the expectations that we have of it. It is not enough for nurses to simply pat themselves on the back for a job well done. We need to understand how we brought about the desirable outcomes. Nurses need to know how to replicate successful care and perhaps then to transfer that to other situations where problems can be solved. As you think about reflection used for this purpose, however, it is necessary to be clear about the criteria used to define success. Do we mean more effective care (greater impact), more efficient care (better use of resources), more sensitive care (working with the needs of patients) or more collegiate care (working better with other professions)?

Correcting practice

Reflection is frequently used to determine what went wrong and what was problematic. *In extremis* it may be used to determine who we believe was to blame for untoward events. Reflection is employed, for instance, as part of a root cause analysis (searching for the origins of a problem) in cases where there are shortfalls in practice or where there has been a near miss (e.g., associated with a drug error) (Carroll, 2009). Reflecting in this way, on what was problematic or erroneous, is taxing. It is emotionally difficult to confront what we believe were our mistakes, and what we might have done better or differently. It becomes more problematic within a blame culture, such as in healthcare where performances are meant to be faultless.

 Reflecting on what seems problematic is often made easier where a mentor is available to assist you. This individual explores with you your perceptions of events and helps you to examine the conclusions that you reach. How big a problem was this? Why did it occur? What were my options? What decisions were important here? What are the pluses as well as the minuses of the course of action that I chose?

Activity 2.4   **Reflection**

Prepare brief points about why, despite the anxieties associated with a blame culture and litigation in healthcare, it remains important for nurses to reflect on what they consider to be their mistakes.

We offer reflections of our own at the end of the chapter.

Understanding self

Authors vary on the extent to which they think reflection should be used to understand ourselves (Bulman and Schutz, 2008; Craig, 2009). In some areas of nursing (e.g., mental health) an understanding of our motives, values and personality is especially important because we use the self to therapeutic purpose. Our ability to share personal insights, or to imagine how others feel, may be critical. Instead of seeing the nurse as someone who musters and applies skills, the nurse is conceived as someone who uses his or her personality as part of therapy. The ability to empathise, for example, becomes integral to entering the world of the patient and their anxieties, but one that must be managed with a certain detachment as well if professional judgements are then to remain sound. A successful mental health nurse builds an excellent rapport with patients and empathises with some of their concerns, but also manages to adopt a position where they can later challenge some of the patients' unhelpful beliefs.

These are important points and may be the focus for some of your concerns as well as some of your later nursing achievements. If you think of nursing in craft terms, your emphasis is likely to be on skills and the ways these are selected and applied. For example, with regard to interpersonal relationships with patients, your reflections may focus on techniques, such as listening, managing silence or clarifying options open to the patient. If, though, you think of nursing in much more vocational and perhaps aesthetic terms, you are likely to feel more comfortable reflecting on your values and beliefs, precisely because you see these as a means to deliver the best care. You are likely to reflect instead on the nature of interpersonal rapport and the accord or otherwise between your own and the patient's values. While the craft-orientated nurse might see such detailed reflection about values, beliefs and motives as somehow intrusive and perhaps even unnecessary, you see these as essential to the development of artful practice.

Activity 2.5	Reflection

Make some brief notes about your personal preferences regarding whether reflection should focus upon our values and beliefs as well as our skills and experiences. If you prefer to reflect at arm's length, consider what happens when we encounter care situations when our deeply seated, and perhaps previously unconsidered, values are strongly contested; for example, when a 60-year-old woman seeks assistance to have a baby.

Conversely, if you habitually like to reflect on values and beliefs, what are the risks if, as a result of this, you start to develop quite strong ideological positions on what nurses should and shouldn't do? What happens if you develop an aversion to protocols that appear to limit the nurse's power to negotiate care priorities, for example?

We offer brief reflections at the end of the chapter, but recommend too that you discuss these matters with a personal tutor.

Understanding others

Much of nursing is concerned with assisting others. Person-centred care is based upon the premise that we can successfully ascertain the patient's needs and aspirations, before taking these into account as part of the care that we agree (McCance et al., 2009). There are some problems, though, with using reflection to understand others and chief among these is what we might call the 'common sense' fallacy. We might take it is a given that people in a particular situation (e.g., when suffering pain) will wish to proceed as we would (to have that pain alleviated). We start to use our preferences and wishes in such situations as something that we believe others will aspire to as well. In the above example, not all patients do aspire to alleviate all of their pain; indeed, some may refuse pain relief measures altogether. A devout Buddhist, for example, might observe that pain has something to teach us and to remove it is unhelpful.

Reflection used to understand others, then, has to be of a more speculative kind and is needed to explore possibilities and ideas that arise out of a situation. The nurse examines their first premises about what the patient was feeling, attempting or dealing with and then rehearses other possibilities that present through reflecting on practice. This is a place where reflection becomes most clearly a part of critical thinking. The nurse reflects not only on that encountered, but also that which could apply there, as in the following example.

Case study: Carl's reflections on Gordon's cardiac rehabilitation

Gordon was well into his cardiac rehabilitation programme and the remedial gymnasts reported that he wasn't making progress. He seemed to hold back from the suggested exercises. Moreover, Gordon wasn't talking much about how things might be when he goes home, a sign perhaps of his uncertainty. But perhaps we have to question the assumption that patients wrap themselves in cotton wool and fear that exercise is too risky. Perhaps they are not all petrified of another heart attack. As I think about this, there seem other possibilities that I need to explore with Gordon. The first of those is that exercise doesn't feature in his lifestyle and that our difficulties are about integrating physical activity into a daily routine. Perhaps, too, there are issues around what Gordon thinks of as being a 'proper patient'. Perhaps being a patient for Gordon is about being cared for, rather than being taught exercise routines. Our hospital could feel more like a college for Gordon right now!

Understanding the profession

It may surprise you to discover that reflection has a part to play in understanding your chosen profession, and there will be opportunities within your course, through debates and seminars as well as through clinical practice, to reflect on what 'nursing is all about'. Such opportunities don't only teach you things, they provide a chance to revisit how nursing seems to change. Part of what sustains you as a practitioner concerns clear ideas about what nurses do, what expertise they bring and what is different about the practice of the nurse. These are important considerations in a healthcare world where nurses are asked to diversify the sorts of work that they engage in (Pearson, 2003; Hek et al., 2004).

Experience offers you a variety of insights into how nursing is seen. For example, in a clinical case conference, you listen to the ways in which different professionals talk about the contribution of nursing. At a lecture, you hear the different debates about the contribution of nursing models to practice. Reflecting at these points involves two things. First, you start to add new pieces of information to your own definition of nursing. Second, you start to understand the extent to which you share the perspectives on nursing propounded by others. This can prompt some uncomfortable feelings as you debate whether you agree with others. Rest assured, though, nursing is a very broad church and it encompasses some very varied positions on what nursing consists of. However passionate another view might seem, there are often opposing views available elsewhere.

Challenging assumptions

We have already briefly referred to the need to challenge assumptions, when we wrote about understanding others above. Reflection plays a major role in changing practice and changing profession over time. Healthcare work isn't static, it evolves incrementally, and what was once seemingly ideal becomes suspect and anachronistic later. For example, if you were to read nursing textbooks from the 1960s, you would discover that nursing care was perceived as a supplemental activity to treatment and that both were often prescribed by the medical consultant in charge. Today, nurses are much more strategic and engage in the design of healthcare and the negotiation of care plans with patients. We have greater autonomy, but also more responsibility.

One of the best uses of reflection is, then, at conference, at study day, or when reading a report or policy associated with nursing, to ascertain whether (a) this reflects your current understanding of best practice, and (b) whether, in the light of what you have encountered there, you need to change. Reflection in this context is often best conducted as part of a group of nurses, and especially where local protocols or best practice guidelines are formulated. Working in concert with others you are more likely to formulate an informed opinion and to counterbalance the first negative emotional response that can arise when you are invited to change. As a student you may have several opportunities to join team meetings and discussion groups where just such reflections are under way.

Making reflection work for you

Having defined reflection and made the case for its importance in nursing, we need to consider next just how you can make reflection work for you. Table 2.1 sets out what we recommend at this stage. We then proceed to examine what is involved in association with each of our recommendations.

There are important points to make with regard to Table 2.1. The first concerns wide-ranging reflection versus purposeful reflection. Some of the frameworks used by students to conduct and record their reflections require of them a review of many issues: what I was trying to do, what happened, what I thought, what I felt, what followed next. This becomes more difficult the more complex the episode of care involved. While these frameworks remind the nurse of the different dimensions of an experience, we still recommend deciding the purpose of reflection as well. Failing to do so may result in you building a series of reflections that are later difficult to use, for example within your professional portfolio. Reflection has a part to play in the demonstration of required course learning outcomes, so at the very least it is important to be able to relate the reflections to these. If you state the purpose of each reflection, you can point to work associated with evaluating, exploring, judging or changing practice.

Students sometimes ask what is the right number of reflections to make and record within a given module or clinical placement. It is a 'how long is a piece of string?' question. What is important with regard to the use of reflections is their quality (something aided by linking each to a purpose) and their fit with the learning outcomes set. It is often better to prepare fewer but more fully developed reflections and those drawn from times when you feel fresh and inquisitive. So much the better if these cover a number of different purposes, helping you to explore the diversity of nursing work.

While some deeply analytical individuals can and do conduct private reflections, the majority benefit from working with a chosen confidante. Clinical placements provide a mentor that you ought to consult, and students are allocated a personal tutor. A good confidante is someone who is willing to take an interest in your experience and learning and who has your trust, even though they sometimes challenge your thinking. Successful confidantes can usually be pictured responding to your reflection: 'yes . . . you could look at it that way and it has these merits. But have you also thought about . . .?'. The confidante helps you to see situations from different perspectives, and to determine what you will observe and think about next.

Table 2.1: First principles of successful reflection.

Recommendation	Notes
Clarify the purpose of your reflection on each occasion that you use it.	However exciting it may seem to reflect freely and openly about events, in practice your thinking will be focused better if you have a stated purpose for the reflection. By asking a question you will scrutinise events more closely, e.g. how did we manage to help that patient control their asthma?
Reflect when you are most ready.	Reflection is often hard work and it may provoke uncomfortable emotions. It is important, then, to select the best times to reflect, when you feel emotionally calm, and where you have found the right space to conduct such work. Reflecting when you are still angry, for instance, will usually produce a record of what was wrong with the situation, rather than about what you have learned yourself.
Identify confidantes with whom you are comfortable reflecting.	While it is possible to reflect on your own, it is also possible to delude yourself about a situation. It is better to reflect with a trusted colleague.
Allocate sufficient time and attention to the enterprise.	Reflection is a meditative activity and it requires as much thinking time as writing time. It is wise to allocate at least 30–60 minutes to produce one or more thoughtful reflections – those that can prove useful later.
Use a reflective framework that works for you and that is accepted by the university.	There is a wide variety of reflective frameworks and some university faculties direct what you should use. You should, though, try to work with one that helps you explore your experiences and thoughts in a way that makes sense to you. If it doesn't, you are less likely to engage in regular reflection.
Create reflective records that you can use again.	To use reflective records later, you need to include enough contextual details to understand the events in question. Make sure that you remind yourself what was happening, when the events occurred and what resources or support were available. Date the record to help you sense any changes in your perspective that occur over time.
In making and using such records, respect the rights of others.	In making reflective records, you necessarily refer to other people, so ensure that you make anonymous their names and roles. It is important to store your records securely and to ensure that you do not unfairly defame others.

As well as thinking about how much time you allocate for reflecting, consider too the sequence of thinking and writing. In part, you are thinking even as you write, but this has the disadvantage that, as your thoughts arrive on the page or the computer screen, further thoughts, sometimes contradictory ones, are triggered. It could be this, it could be that. This was important, but then again perhaps it wasn't. Therefore it seems beneficial to allow yourself thinking-only time, or perhaps 'think and scribble ideas down' time, so that you can play with the possibilities before you. It is worth remembering that, while the final written reflection doesn't necessarily need to be highly polished, it should be sufficiently accessible and coherent so that you can use it to revise care later. For that reason, it is our practice to think and draft thoughts first and then to pen reflective records for further use once we have completed the first explorations of the experience. Both spontaneous scribbles and final reflections can be recorded in your portfolio if you wish (offering a full audit trail of thought).

Activity 2.6   *Research*

If you have not already done so, investigate which reflective framework is recommended in association with your course. Discuss with your tutor what is expected in association with each of the headings there, and whether the course permits any latitude with regard to how you set out your records. Establish whether the framework recommended allows you to state clearly the purpose of your reflection, or whether you need to add this as a preliminary introduction.

As this activity is based on your own experience, there is no answer at the end of the chapter.

CHAPTER SUMMARY

We have now reached the end of your introduction to reflection. In this chapter we have suggested that reflection is a form of critical thinking – one that focuses in particular upon experience and that takes into account the emotions associated with experience as well as an account of empirical events. In practice, reflection seems like two skills in one. If we reflect in action, we are thinking on our feet and reading practice situations as quickly and as accurately as possible. If we reflect on action, we use the benefits of hindsight but need to beware that reflecting too long after an event can result in problems associated with memory. By practising both skills you will become better equipped to use experience to professional advantage, to understand how your perceptions relate to others, and to appreciate how this can then improve your understanding of your work as a nurse. While it is unrealistic to analyse all experiences in situ (you would suffer from information overload), it is possible to accumulate reflections after events, increasing your insights into your motives, actions and the consequences of what you do.

Reflection, however, involves a process and several activities, for example deciding when to reflect, identifying a purpose, choosing how to frame the reflection and making a record. In support of that, we have shared a series of what we suggest are best principles associated with this work. It is important here to work with university reflective frameworks. This is because reflection is itself a part of the curriculum and the ways in which students are expected to learn.

Activities: brief outline answers and reflections

Activity 2.2: Critical thinking (page 25)

We suggest that perception plays a major part in healthcare. Patients perceive nurses in particular ways and then carry assumptions about what nursing care will be like. Similarly, we carry our own assumptions about patients and care team colleagues. The point is, however, that perceptions consist of sensory information (what we see, hear or smell) and our interpretation of those sensations. The latter is usually informed by past experiences, education and upbringing, so in thinking about reflection we need to be cautious about perceptions. Our perceptions could be subject to bias, prejudice or cultural limitations that limit our understanding of what is going on around us. One of the key reasons for reflecting with a confidante, or for sharing our notes with others, is to overcome some of the limitations that perception can pose.

Historically, nurses have tended to reflect using frameworks that emphasised a wide-ranging review of different aspects of experience. This seems an important first step, but we argue that the records obtained in this way don't deepen our analysis of experience. It is difficult to be 'critically reflective' unless we approach reflection in a more purposeful way. We hope you agree that reflection is a rich and rewarding activity, but one that benefits from a clear purpose.

Activity 2.4: Reflection (page 27)

There are a number of good reasons to reflect. Among the ones that we noted were:

- being professional (we need to examine what we do);
- resolving problems and discomforts (reflection can help us manage the stress associated with practice);
- personal growth and skill development (much of what we do requires practice insights, and these aren't readily obtained from research or a textbook);
- understanding our own position or perspective (we are less likely to feel angry or frustrated if we understand why our position is different from that of others).

Activity 2.5: Reflection (page 28)

Our discussions revealed that one of the authors of this book, Bob Price, sees reflection working more in association with skills and that the other, Anne Harrington, sees reflection as working in more personal value terms. The positions are not in complete opposition, though, because we agree that care cannot proceed without an under-standing of both skills, and values and beliefs. It is just that we feel differently about how far reflection might take us in each of these areas! Bob conceives of the nurse as a skilful craftsperson, in some instances a master craftsperson of nursing care. Skills are central to his notion of nursing. Anne conversely sees nursing in more vocational terms, as something that works very closely with the personality of the practitioner. Professional care is an accentuation of human care – that which we intuitively subscribe to. Happily, both have their place.

Knowledge review

Having worked through this chapter, rate your understanding of the following topics as one of the following: poor, adequate, improving or excellent.

1. The differences between reflecting in action and on action, including the challenges associated with each.
2. The definition of reflection.
3. The different purposes to which reflection can be put.
4. Best practice principles that will ensure reflection works well for you.

Make a short (and dated) note about whether you feel comfortable about the prospect of reflecting on events with others. We recommend that you revisit these notes again after you have finished reading this book. Attitudes towards reflection can and do shift!

Further reading

Bulman, C and Schutz, S (2008) *Reflective Practice in Nursing*, 4th edition. Oxford: Blackwell.
A wide-ranging discussion of reflective practice and the merits of reflection in a profession that deals with patients' experiences and emotions as well as their injuries and illness.

Jasper, M (2003) *Foundations in Nursing and Health Care: Beginning reflective practice.* Cheltenham: Nelson Thornes.
Melanie Jasper is at her strongest writing about journaling and what this adds to learning. An established resource.

Johns, C (2004) *Becoming a Reflective Practitioner*, 2nd edition. London: Wiley Blackwell.
One of several authors who have suggested frameworks for the organisation of reflection.

Useful websites

www.practicebasedlearning.org/resources/materials/intro.htm
Allin, L and Turnock, C (2007) *Reflection On and In the Workplace for Work-based Supervisors*, Making Practice-Based Learning Work.
While this website is not specifically aimed at nurses, it provides a useful review of different aspects of reflection and reflective practice, including the document above, with a special emphasis on work-based reflection. There are items on making reflective records and what mentors can do to aid reflection. A simple and accessible addition to your reading.

Chapter 3

Scholarly writing

NMC Standards for Pre-registration Nursing Education (2010)

This chapter will address the following competencies.

Domain: Communication and interpersonal skills

3. All nurses must use the full range of communication methods, including verbal, non-verbal and written, to acquire, interpret and record their knowledge and understanding of people's needs. They must be aware of their own values and beliefs and the impact this may have on their communication with others. They must take account of the many different ways in which people communicate and how these may be influenced by ill health, disability and other factors, and be able to recognise and respond effectively when a person finds it hard to communicate.
7. All nurses must maintain accurate, clear and complete records, including the use of electronic formats, using appropriate and plain language.

Domain: Leadership, management and team working

2. All nurses must systematically evaluate care and ensure that they and others use the findings to help improve people's experience and care outcomes and to shape future services.

Chapter aims

By the end of this chapter you will be able to:

- summarise what we mean by scholarly writing;
- discuss the key features of essay structure and how these facilitate your explanation of learning achieved to date;
- explore the ways in which past experiences of writing can shape assumptions about academic writing in the future;
- make a clear case for 'thinking time' when preparing to write an academic paper;
- identify areas within your own writing where there is future scope for development.

Introduction

We start this chapter with three observations that we hope reassure you. First, writing in a scholarly way seems to us a relatively new skill for most students. This means that what we think of as the 'craftwork of writing' deserves help and support. Even though you may have written academic essays at school, it is less likely that these will also have been vocational works, that is, papers written about a practice such as nursing. Second, writing in a scholarly way can be successfully learned provided that you take a little time to consider the process of work before you. While there are several different writing formats used within most nursing courses (e.g., writing reflectively, writing about theory, writing plans and reports), all are open to analysis and students can and do improve their writing with practice. We return to different formats of writing in the third part of this book. Third, the writing skills you learn here will serve you well for the rest of your career. You will be surprised just how often they are used in the future, whether that is in association with courses of study, writing for publication or perhaps preparing reports associated with your work as a nurse.

Stewart, Fatima, Raymet and Gina (the four students you met in Chapter 1) support the contentions shared here, but it won't surprise you that, like other students, they sometimes find writing difficult. Stewart came to nursing from a career in commerce, where his writing was much more sparing and less reflective than is often required in nursing. Fatima and Raymet note that they not only wrestle with writing in the required nursing form, but also with some of the conventions of academic discussion as presented in British universities. There were different traditions of writing where they studied before, in India and Botswana, where their schooling focused on writing about factual knowledge and was less philosophical than is often required in nursing. Gina thinks that she starts with the clearest possible start point, as she is not used to any other tradition in writing. She has the most recent experience of secondary education, but she does not feel this has equipped her for the higher level and applied nature of nursing programmes. She also feels she lacks the life experience of the others to draw on in her writing, which is often required in nursing. Their personal tutors have acknowledged the various challenges they all face, observing that students who move between one career, culture or educational system and another need help to adapt to the expectations of their new environment. It is not that new ways of reasoning or writing are inherently superior, but that they dictate the ways in which assessors review pieces of coursework and examination scripts. Within a course of nursing studies, there may be many different forms of writing required – that which is reflective, analytical or strategic in nature. Irrespective of which background students come from, then, new skills will have to be learned and past assumptions about writing reconsidered. Conventions of reasoning and writing in the university where the student studies now, and those that guide judgements about good work there, need to be understood if students are to succeed. This includes supporting the development of graduate-level academic writing skills.

In this chapter we will be working with the experiences of Stewart and his colleagues, and leading you through different aspects of scholarly writing. Importantly, that involves the connection of critical thinking and reflection to the conventions of scholarly discourse. We will examine the ways in which you might best represent what you have reasoned and reflected upon. First, we examine how best to prepare for writing. Second, we turn to the basic structure of academic pieces of work. While this will vary, dependent upon the format of writing that you are asked to engage in, we believe that there are some opening tenets of good writing that can be learned here. Lastly, we discuss what we mean by 'academic voice'. We use this term based on the research of the first of the authors of this book, where it was discovered that students need to understand the way in which they wish to present their learning to others (Price, 2003b). Sometimes we need to convey what others have discovered, and sometimes we need to convey our own philosophy, but most often we need to write to very disciplined purpose, demonstrating our command of the teaching provided. The clearer you are about academic voice, the better able you will be to link learning to written work.

Activity 3.1   *Reflection*

Take a moment now to think about your background in writing, the strengths and the challenges that you think you have concerning your writing to date, and the writing that may be required on your course.

- Are you like Stewart, accomplished in another writing tradition but uncertain about the nursing one?
- Are you like Fatima and Raymet, used to writing in other ways associated with another educational system?
- Do you share something with Gina in that you wonder whether a lack of experience may disadvantage you?
- Perhaps you are different, rich with life experience, but it has been a long time since you studied and you worry that your writing will seem 'rusty'?

Setting notes down now will help you understand the work ahead better.

As this activity is based on your own reflection, there is no answer at the end of the chapter.

Preparing to write

Students are surprised by the emphasis that we place upon preparation time, imagining that we compose as we write. In our experience, though, there is real benefit in allocating 'thinking time' before you write. This is not simply a matter of making a plan, it is about distilling your thoughts before you try to use them to represent your learning. Tutors regularly comment that they can see in academic essays where students are thinking as they write. Problems then include:

- not answering the question set, or preparing the wrong sort of coursework;
- allocating the word count poorly within the essay (early sections getting the lion's share of attention and later sections suffering);
- material being presented in an incompletely reasoned state (it is hard to go back and edit an essay when you fear that, in doing so, you may lose the plot and write something inferior);
- essay conclusions falling short of requirement, because students have argued many things but have never quite determined what they think.

We asked our students to each consider one of the preparations in Figure 3.1 that we think of as important in scholarly writing. Your challenge in turn is to identify the opportunities that you have to engage in such preparatory work. Where do your opportunities exist to think about an academic essay in preparation?

Our own illustrations are summarised at the end of the chapter.

Coming from a different professional background, Stewart is already attuned to the need to understand the writing task set. Nursing courses include a wide variety of forms of writing and each is closely associated with reasoning in different ways. For example, if you are asked to present a portfolio of learning, you will need to write reflectively but also include elements of strategy as you present plans for developing your work in the future. We suggest, therefore, that you not only read the requirements carefully (the assignment brief, the report required by a manager, etc.), but that you take time to clarify any concerns and queries with the person who set the brief.

Many of you may empathise with Fatima's response about the difficulty of adopting a position within a piece of coursework. In the past, students have often been required to summarise what others have said, especially teachers. Past courses may have been more pedagogical, and assign the teacher a greater role, confirming either what can fairly be supported, or what is most acceptable. In yet others, teachers have more of a facilitation role, and are charged with prompting the students to work through issues to reach their own conclusions. The move from a background where teaching was more prominent, to

Figure 3.1

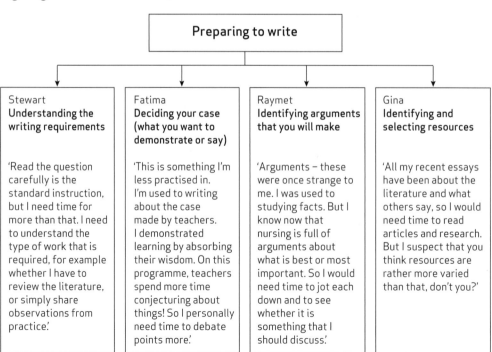

Preparing to write

Stewart
Understanding the writing requirements

'Read the question carefully is the standard instruction, but I need time for more than that. I need to understand the type of work that is required, for example whether I have to review the literature, or simply share observations from practice.'

Fatima
Deciding your case (what you want to demonstrate or say)

'This is something I'm less practised in. I'm used to writing about the case made by teachers. I demonstrated learning by absorbing their wisdom. On this programme, teachers spend more time conjecturing about things! So I personally need time to debate points more.'

Raymet
Identifying arguments that you will make

'Arguments – these were once strange to me. I was used to studying facts. But I know now that nursing is full of arguments about what is best or most important. So I would need time to jot each down and to see whether it is something that I should discuss.'

Gina
Identifying and selecting resources

'All my recent essays have been about the literature and what others say, so I would need time to read articles and research. But I suspect that you think resources are rather more varied than that, don't you?'

one where the facilitation of learning predominates, is difficult for students (Cortazzi and Jinn, 1997), so don't worry if you are finding the transition hard! In our experience, this is heightened in many areas of the nursing curriculum, where students are required to 'adopt a position', to 'take a stance on an issue' of their own. For example, in rehabilitation, where work is shared with patients and lay carers, you might be asked to state what represents a reasonable level of support. What do you expect patients or relatives to learn and do, and what do you think we as nurses should contribute? In these and similar matters, you do need to make a case and it is then important for you to be completely clear about this before you start. It takes time to discover and settle on your position before writing.

Raymet's points are important: students often wonder when an argument becomes a fact! Moreover, if you are to grapple with a series of arguments, how should they best be arranged? In nursing courses, there is often a need to present a series of arguments, each of which supports the case or position that we adopt. You will often find within UK universities that the case or position is stated early within the academic paper and the main text is then used to rehearse arguments and counter arguments, which help the student to sum up insights within their conclusion (there are other approaches within reflective writing that we explore elsewhere). In our example, your case or position may be that nurses should educate patients to take on self-care activities. Arguments in support of this then include (a) that patients gain independence through their own learning, (b) that it is not economically viable to go on delivering all the care, so patients and relatives need to develop their own skills, and (c) that patients develop greater self-esteem through the process of learning to self-care. This may or may not be your experience of previous learning, where perhaps you revealed your position incrementally at the end of your paper. However, the case-first sequence is the reasoning norm for more philosophical essays within nursing, so if you have difficulties making that transition it is worth discussing the adjustments that you are trying to make with your personal tutor.

Gina is correct that we envisage students using a variety of resources as part of their academic writing and that it takes time to select what will be included in a piece of coursework. Observations from practice, arguments articulated by others in interview, and hospital care philosophies are just a few of the things that could support what you write about. It takes time to evaluate each of these and to judge how each resource will be linked to the arguments made (*this* supports my argument, *that* reminds us there are alternative perspectives).

Activity 3.3   *Reflection*

Look back now to your answers to Activity 3.1 and decide, in the light of your notes made there, what is now important about *your* preparation for writing. Will you need to understand the assignment question or task better because you share a background similar to Stewart's? Like Raymet, will it be helpful to speak to your tutor in order to understand whether you have prepared a clear case and well-developed arguments within a planned paper?

As this activity is based on your own reflection, there is no answer at the end of the chapter.

The basics of structure

While academic coursework varies according to what form of writing is required, several tenets of good academic structure are worth remembering. Pieces of academic work have a beginning, a middle and an end and must seem complete and coherent. It is this quality of completeness and coherence, together with authority, clarity and precision, that we search for when planning a paper. Completeness and coherence are supported by the way in which we structure the coursework, authority is determined by how we present and support arguments, and clarity and precision are affected by how we help others to navigate the paper, and through the way in which we decide what to include and what to leave out. Force too much information into an essay and clarity suffers.

Activity 3.4   *Research*

To help you to explore structure more fully, we have included an analytical essay within the *Learning Matters* website (**www.learningmatters.co.uk/nursing**). Studying this will help you examine the points that we make below. If you do not have access to the web, or if the site is temporarily unavailable, you may prefer instead to examine an article published within a nursing journal. If you choose this second option, we recommend that you select an article that explores a topic (e.g., rehabilitation nursing), rather than one that reports research. While published works are more polished than those submitted for coursework assessment, they nevertheless include relevant structural features that we can discuss.

When you have selected a resource, refer to it and answer our questions at the end of each of the following sections.

As this activity, and those following, depend on the resource you have chosen, there are no answers given for the remaining activities in this chapter.

Introducing the work

All pieces of academic work need an introduction and this has four roles:

- to identify the subject matter of the piece written;
- to secure the readers' attention and interest;
- to establish the writer's position or perspective;
- to set any contexts that the paper needs to be understood within.

It is possible to establish the subject matter by stating the essay question set or to simply say at the outset, 'This essay is written about the rehabilitation work of the nurse.' However, there are slightly more adventurous ways of introducing a subject. An academic essay is not journalism, but like journalists we are required to interest our readers in the essay subject matter, even if they are examiners and are paid to read our work! We need a 'hook' to encourage them to read on. Two common ways to do that are to either:

- start with a bold point – one that highlights the importance of the subject matter, for example: 'There is at least anecdotal evidence that nurses and patients are not always working to the same ends, regarding rehabilitation';

or

- introduce a dilemma that needs to be addressed – for example: 'There is a problem with patient rehabilitation and this is linked to what we consider ideal and what seems possible given resource constraints.'

You will need to decide whether your introduction will be presented in first person singular (referring to 'I') or in third person, referring to 'the nurse' or 'nurses'. First person singular is increasingly the norm where any form of reflective writing is required. Where in third person you refer to 'the author', it is important to beware of literature review traps. Are you talking about the author of other papers reviewed, or you, the author of this essay?

If your work concerns practice or an area of professional discourse (e.g., applied science or pharmacology), your introduction needs to make this clear. You might, for instance, refer to a client group that your work concerns (such as post-operative patients) or a particular area of practice (e.g., the use of analgesia).

Activity 3.5	Reflection

Examine now your chosen essay or article in order to establish whether the introduction achieves all of these things. If any of the key features are missing, what are the implications for the rest of the piece?

Signposting the work

Towards the end of the introduction to your work, you need to help the reader understand how the rest of the work is set out ('This essay is set out in the following sections . . .'). Signposting is not only a description of the rest of the work, though; it frequently includes an indication of the stance that you take and the purpose of your paper. You may indicate that this paper on rehabilitation nursing considers the role of the nurse in section 1, and the role of patients and lay carers in section 2, and then debates the liaison work between the two groups in section 3 ('The paper makes the case that rehabilitation is a negotiated activity and one that requires careful liaison between stakeholders').

Activity 3.6	Critical thinking

Did you spot signposting in the work that you chose to read? It frequently consists of just one very important paragraph at the end of the introduction. Does the signposting within your reviewed work help you read forward with a clear purpose, knowing what the author is trying to do?

Developing the main body of the work

Classically, academic essays include a main text that has few subsections and that rarely includes figures or tables. Within nursing, however, the conventions are rapidly changing and it is usual to arrange the work using subheadings that help the reader to navigate your work, and both figures and tables where these help you to make a point quickly and clearly. We suggest that you check your course handbook to establish what the local norms are. Our own preference is to encourage writing that helps the reader to follow your arguments, and that includes features that are similar to those used when writing for publication (section headings and tables or figures).

What remains important in academic papers is that you write in disciplined paragraphs, that you write short sentences that enable you to make clear points, and that where you do use figures, tables or appendices, these are all clearly referred to in the text and within brackets (e.g., 'see Figure 1', 'Table 3 refers', 'see Appendix 1').

What do we mean by a disciplined paragraph? In practical terms it is one that:

- attends to a single subject (e.g., ascertaining the patient's readiness to rehabilitate);
- includes clear points, your own or others' arguments (e.g., 'While economic pressures exist to speed up rehabilitation, the readiness of a patient to learn skills remains important');
- provides support for what has been stated. This is often where references to the literature come in, but as we have noted, other evidence gleaned from practice could be referred to (e.g., 'An example patient helps to make the case. Mr X reported that he felt paralysed by fear regarding taking exercise after his heart attack. He worried that staff had not completely understood the risks').

Sentences that extend beyond a couple of lines of text are much more likely to seem ambiguous to the reader. Being scholarly does not necessarily mean writing longer sentences, or cramming more information into a paragraph!

These presentation points accepted, the last key consideration regarding the main text is that you build a series of arguments there. To demonstrate that you are thinking critically, it is important not to accept points at face value. For this reason, a paragraph that makes one argument could, in some instances, be followed by another paragraph that makes a second argument. But it is important by the end of your work to demonstrate that you have reached your own conclusions, even if this is only to suggest that the debate continues. Turning once more to our example, we might spend one paragraph arguing the above point about the importance of patients' readiness to commence rehabilitation, and then add a second that reminds the reader that prolonged inactivity increases the risk of post-myocardial infarction complications. On balance, then, the recommended way forward is physical rehabilitation and consistent psychological support while patients test their limits.

Activity 3.7   *Critical thinking*

Examine your chosen essay or article now, in order to identify some examples of what you think are especially successful paragraphs and to list the arguments that you can see being developed within the main text of the paper. How does this structure compare with some of your own past essays? Can you see how the work starts to have a bigger impact on you because of its structure?

Reaching a conclusion

Academic coursework (unless otherwise instructed) requires a conclusion. Within the conclusion there should be no substantially new material. The purpose of the conclusion is to sum up what has been written so far. However, the essay has to show what sense has been made about the arguments presented. Beyond all those points about helping the patient rehabilitate, what does all this amount to? The author needs to deduce what the arguments support. Perhaps it is first to support patients, because they are doing a lot of the rehabilitation work. Perhaps it is to coordinate rehabilitation work. Perhaps it is that if physiotherapy is given before patient education has been delivered patient anxiety might be increased.

Activity 3.8   *Critical thinking*

Scrutinise your chosen paper to see whether the conclusion achieves the above. Don't be surprised if you identify some shortfalls here. Even published papers sometimes include weak conclusions. Did the conclusion make reference to a case that was stated at the start of the essay or article?

Adopting the right voice

We come at last to the business of 'voice'. You might be surprised that we use a term more associated with singing to describe scholarly writing. By voice we mean conveying your thoughts in such a way that your thinking is demonstrated as something that seems orderly, measured, critical or reflective, as the need dictates. Singers use a voice to convey emotions or drama. Students need, through their texts, to use a voice to illustrate or represent their learning. We have already conveyed two ways in which your work will seem more scholarly – the first developing a coherent structure for your work, and the second building a series of arguments that demonstrate your reasoning. There remain, though, some important niceties in the ways in which you write (use your voice) that will enhance your reputation as a scholar.

Activity 3.9   *Critical thinking*

Look now at some sample sentences that our four students used in their earliest essays. They are at pains to remind us that their work has improved since! There are some classic faults within these short extracts that demonstrate less than scholarly work, and we now invite you to identify them.

Gina: 'That patients wait, lying on trolleys within a corridor or a corner of Casualty, is utterly appalling.'
Stewart: 'Time is money, so the doctor's stay at the bedside is always short and patients ask others what has then been decided as regards their treatment.'
Raymet: 'The assessment I made of the patient was holistic. I examined their rash and listened carefully to their anxieties.'
Fatima: 'A tutor has explained that patients sometimes only want to please the nurse, rather than state their real concerns. This seems right to me.'

We wonder whether you spotted the fact that Gina was using hyperbole; that is, accentuating a point made in a heavy-handed or excessive way. While we might share dismay at the length of time patients wait to secure a bed, and wouldn't commend long waiting times and uncomfortable conditions, the conventions of academic writing are that we express opinion in rather more measured terms. In this example, a more measured critique of this situation might be to observe that the lengthy waits were undignified, that they brought into question the adequacy of resources, and that they raised questions about service standards. The phrase 'utterly appalling' appeals to the emotions of the reader rather than their intellect, and we don't convey analysis so clearly. A scholarly voice is measured – one where the writer does not move easily and quickly to emotional condemnation or superlatives ('the care was fantastic') for example when praising practice in another.

Stewart's fault in this example concerned what we call a colloquialism – that is, a form of shorthand writing that we assume the reader understands. 'Time is money' is a well-known aphorism that describes how people prioritise their time using economic considerations. But used in this context it hardly does justice to the doctor. There is certainly a problem here, because patients may need lengthy explanations of planned treatment, but this is a problem of time and resources and says something too about information-sharing and informed consent. 'Time is money' does not do justice to the matter and conveys (the unintended) message that some matters are obvious and can quickly be dismissed in an academic essay.

The fault in Raymet's writing is rather more subtle, but nonetheless a good example of where the scholarly voice has not yet been developed. If work is to be precise, it is necessary to use terms and concepts with care. In this instance, Raymet is referring to holism and claiming that the assessment of a patient was holistic. However, holistic refers to four major aspects of a person's life and experience: the physical, the psychological, the social and the spiritual. It suggests that the care delivered engages deeply and comprehensively with the patient's experience (Brooker and Waugh, 2007). What Raymet reports here is not a holistic assessment of the patient, but one that concentrates upon the rash (physical) and patient anxieties (psychological). No mention is made of spiritual concerns or social needs. It is important, then, to use terms precisely. Checking a dictionary can help to resolve this issue.

There are two possible problems with the academic voice in Fatima's extract. First, there are usually conventions associated with the referencing of sources and here Fatima is not following them. If she has been encouraged to include personal discourses with a tutor within academic work, it is necessary to state in brackets the nature of that (e.g., 'personal email communication with tutor X'). Second, students sometimes present work that is designed to please a tutor or other marker of the finished work. They may refer with approval to what the examiner has taught, said or written elsewhere. In scholarly writing, though, examiners wish to learn what the student has reasoned rather than what the tutor has taught. It is necessary to demonstrate your own judgement and evaluation of issues, rather than to simply approve those that you think might please someone else.

Thus, a scholarly voice is one that:

- acknowledges the source of points and/or perspectives of others (in the literature or elsewhere);
- demonstrates your own reasoning and reflection;
- uses terms precisely and consistently;
- expresses points in a measured rather than an emotive way;
- avoids forms of shorthand reasoning such as colloquialisms.

C H A P T E R   S U M M A R Y

We will return to the matter of scholarly writing again in Part 3 of this book, and especially the differences that happen when you write reflectively. It is important here, however, to acknowledge the above precepts of good writing, some of which can seem implicit rather than explained within the course that you study. Pausing to consider what is required of you by your tutor and the university, and where that fits and doesn't fit with what you have learned before, can help you to understand what seems more challenging about study. Most of what is required is determined by the need to convey your learning in as clear and accessible a manner as possible: by adhering to simple practices, by writing a paper that has a clear beginning, middle and end, and by using devices to guide the reader through the work. It is about considering how much information you can or should include within a sentence or paragraph, and whether your work within that paragraph has strayed away from its subject. It is certainly about good spelling and grammar, as well as checking work before it is submitted. These are precepts we assume you have accepted and used in courses prior to university.

Of all the fundamental errors in scholarship writing that we see within nurse education programmes, there are three that recur frequently. Some students fail to appreciate what sort of writing they are asked to provide. Like Stewart, they need to clarify the requirements set, usually by taking questions to the tutor. Other students begin to write long before they have concluded what they think. They are then hard pressed to identify what case they wish to present. 'Thinking time' is more important than 'writing time' and it is worth investing in, especially if you jot down notes about your developing ideas. A third group of students rush forward with their writing, failing to attend to the academic voice required within assignments. They use imprecise colloquial terms. The net effect is that their work seems ill considered and hurriedly prepared. Many of the papers that students have criticised as 'too descriptive' are associated with such faults. Arguments are lacking and the ideas discussed have been handled in a shorthand way.

Examining examples of scholarly writing in different places will help you to identify what conveys learning clearly and well. By studying the resources associated with this chapter, or those that you find within the university library, you will be much better placed to represent your reasoning and reflection when it comes to work that carries course marks.

Activities: brief outline answers and reflections

Activity 3.2: Critical thinking (page 38)

Preparation is everything! Most of the assessment requirements of a module are set out within the course handbook – so there is significant scope to read, reread and ask questions about the nature of the writing required. It is extremely unwise to leave questions about coursework assessment requirements until the last few days before an assignment is due for submission.

The development of your case (on a given topic) occurs incrementally and may be associated with your reading on the module, the discussions you have within your tutorial group, and perhaps the reflections that you share during a clinical placement. This is where note-taking comes in. You are most likely to develop clear ideas if you jot down observations on a theme that is important for your assessment. What did you note from the lecture or the discussion group? What does your clinical placement mentor have to say about the subject? What did you notice in a textbook that you read? These are all things that help you to think about what others think and where you stand on a subject, before you get to an essay submission.

Arguments are also developed in association with your reading, listening and reflecting. If you take up position X, what supports this position? What makes the position that you take rather more difficult to sustain? We remember some heated discussions associated with the extended role of the nurse and whether, as a result, some caring skills were swopped for technical or medical skills. Was there scope for continuing to listen in the same way, to empathise so effectively and to explore needs, while performing a greater array of technical skills? Rehearsing what seemed possible, in our experience, enabled us to advance arguments about whether nurses should or should not extend their practice.

Lessons, workshops, discussion groups and set reading are also places where we have found resources to support essays. It is important to decide what fits and what doesn't with a given essay, but it is surprising just what might help you to make a case. Consider, for example, our discussion at the start of Chapter 2 as to whether TV reality shows tell us something useful about reflection. Do you agree with us that they help to explain a natural instinct to reflect and to judge? Do you think that, in turn, they help us to exercise caution in jumping to premature conclusions?

Knowledge review

It is time now to take stock of your discoveries associated with this chapter. Consider whether each of the following is still unfamiliar, partially mastered (understood in significant part) or mastered.

1. The basic structure of an academic essay (variants will be discussed in Part 3).
2. The different ways in which your past study, or traditions of learning and writing, can either support or undermine what is needed within academic writing now.
3. The markers of what counts as scholarly work (e.g., the use of measured terms).

If you discovered a lot that is only 'partially mastered' in this review don't be too disheartened. Students start from different points and places along this journey. The clearer you are about outstanding challenges, the better you are equipped to improve your writing in the future. Knowing what you wish to ask a tutor about helps a great deal.

Further reading

By definition, we see a niche need for a book on reasoning, reflecting and writing in nursing (this one). There are, however, two other texts that we admire on the more general principles of essay writing. You would do well to look at these, if you wish to augment your reading of our chapters.

Hennessey, B (2008) *Writing An Essay: Simple techniques to transform your coursework and examinations*, 5th edition. Oxford: How to Books.
This is an accessible guide to the general principles of good writing and the marshalling of information within an essay.

Warburton, N (2006) *The Basics of Essay Writing*. Oxford: Routledge.
This is equally good, focusing additionally on the psychology of planning an essay and deciding when best to stop thinking and start writing.

Useful websites

www.surrey.ac.uk/Skills/pack/essay.html
Communications: Essay writing, University of Surrey
Most universities supply their own guide on good writing practice, but this site offers an especially good stepwise guide, with bullet points that you can check as you prepare, compose and later review your work.

A very important note

Any internet search using the phrase 'essay writing' will draw your attention to a large number of firms, who for a fee will write essays on a student's behalf. To use these, presenting others' work as your own within coursework assessment, is likely to lead to disciplinary measures being taken against you, both by the university and perhaps by the Nursing and Midwifery Council. If you cheat in this way, you run the risk of damaging your career. You will learn little unless you work with bona fide textbooks and tutors to develop your written work skills. The latter are needed throughout a nursing career, so short cutting the skill to pass an assessment achieves little. Later requirements in practice will expose what has not been learnt. Universities have sophisticated systems for spotting plagiarism and regularly monitor submissions, comparing these against past student work and that sold by internet-based essay writing companies.

Part 2

Critical thinking and reflecting in nursing contexts

Chapter 4

Making sense of lectures

NMC Standards for Pre-registration Nursing Education (2010)

Because the subject matter of lectures varies widely, there are no specific standards to link to. The skills covered in this chapter underpin how you successfully learn and achieve all the standards, within the environment of lectures.

Chapter aims

By the end of this chapter you will be able to:

- detail ways to engage in the lecture so as to enhance the quality of your learning;
- summarise ways in which to prepare for a lecture;
- discuss the different ways of thinking in a lecture that might enrich your experience;
- explain why questions are so important to learning in a lecture;
- summarise important things to do after the lecture has ended.

Introduction

Nursing courses provide a range of learning opportunities, each of which enables you to discuss ideas with others and explore issues that may have arisen through what you see and hear. Among those learning opportunities, lectures make a major contribution. Lectures are well suited to conveying significant amounts of information to large numbers of students and can, in skilful hands, convey a great deal about how the nurse reasons (Race, 2007). Lectures are delivered in subject areas such as anatomy and physiology, pharmacology, nursing theory, healthcare ethics and nursing management. Accomplished lecturers admit you into their own thought processes and help you to explore the possibilities that they consider. You gain insight into how a tutor weighs the pros and cons of issues, and determines what is of higher priority or most significant in caring for patients. Because, in most instances, tutors talk more than students within the lecture, there is a risk that your approach to learning could be unduly passive. It is possible, for instance, to attend a lecture and to gain comparatively little from it, not necessarily because the lecture was poorly delivered, but because you did not focus inquisitively enough on what was shared.

It is crucial that you gain the most from those lectures that you attend, especially where the subject is not repeated later and subsequent teaching assumes that a subject has been grasped. If you miss such opportunities, your future learning may be impaired and you might fail related assessments. The better organised you are as regards learning in lectures, the more you will derive from them.

In this chapter, we assist you to plan for forthcoming lectures and to arrive at each in an inquisitive state of mind. We describe the features of typical lectures and identify how best to arrive at a balance between listening, thinking, writing and communicating. In particular, we attend to learning associated with questions in the lecture – those that the tutor might pose to you and those that, in turn, you might want to ask. We finish the chapter with some work that you should undertake after the lecture has ended.

Activity 4.1   *Reflection*

No one supposes that every lecture is perfect. However, to help you to orientate discussions within this chapter, begin now by recalling a particularly successful lecture that you enjoyed. Identify what seemed to make the lecture such a success. Was success determined largely by the skills of the tutor, the contributions of the students, or a mixture of the two?

At the end of the chapter we summarise some features of memorable lectures that we have attended and highlight the part played by students.

Preparing for the lecture

Every lecture that you attend has the potential to enhance your thinking, and to develop further your confidence as a nurse. However, it is not necessarily the case that you will let it. There are all sorts of potential barriers to successful learning in lectures and some of them are associated with our assumptions and expectations. We may come to the lecture anxious that we will not grasp the subject material, perhaps because this subject seemed difficult in the past. We might already have decided that the subject is dull and, in our view at least, even irrelevant. Rather arrogantly, we might assume that we have already mastered the subject matter and see this as a lecture 'more for those who didn't study this subject previously'. Lectures don't pan out exactly as we expect, though. If we are open to new ideas, we discover something fresh, challenging, interesting and reassuring within most of them.

To illustrate this, imagine the scene where students who hold the assumptions listed in Table 4.1 encounter some rather exciting lectures.

The purpose of Table 4.1 is to highlight how assumptions about a lecture can serve either to enhance or to undermine your learning. If you were the first student, attending a lecture on schizophrenia, you might be delighted to discover that the tutor has adopted such an imaginative approach, introducing you to schizophrenia from the patient's point of view. This is not the usual stance adopted within textbooks. But you will have been jolted from your anticipated line of thought – one that catalogued the signs, symptoms and theories about the condition. Entering this lecture with rigidly set ideas about what will happen next could leave you needing to adjust during the first ten minutes of the

Table 4.1: Student expectations and lecture encounters.

Lecture subject matter	Student expectation	Lecture format
Understanding mental illness: an introduction to schizophrenia	This lecture will augment what I have read in a textbook (so is not that valuable).	The lecturer uses a series of audiotapes that first simulate what it is like for patients to 'hear voices' and to suffer delusional thoughts, before discussing a videotape of a patient talking about coping with this.
Risk assessment and management in clinical areas	This is important stuff, but I guess it will list what we have to do, and what we must control or avoid (it will instruct).	The lecturer confronts the audience with a story of a 'near miss' drug error and casts them as fellow investigators in what needs to be done next.
A physiology lesson on endocrine control of the body	I have studied physiology at college before and can list all the important endocrine organs and hormones.	The lecturer presents complex information from the start of the lecture. Each student is provided with an electronic device that they can press to indicate when they don't understand something. Lights relating to this show up on the lectern that the lecturer speaks from. The lecturer proceeds apace, provided that lights do not go on in front of him.

presentation. Perhaps some important points are then missed during this adjustment period. If you were the second student, you might have been surprised to find that you were cast in the role of fellow incident investigator. The tutor punctuates her lecture with a series of questions to the audience: 'What might we do here?' 'Why do you think this important?' If you were the third student, your view of your own understanding of endocrinology may have been tested, but will you press the button to indicate when you don't understand something that has been said by the tutor? The discomfort of discovering what you really don't know, and thought that you did, may mean that you are reluctant to signal to the lecturer that he is covering ground too quickly.

The key point here is that lectures do more than simply convey information. Tutors have become more artful about lecture format, so you need to engage much more carefully with what is shared. The best way to prepare mentally for lectures, then, is to acknowledge in advance your misgivings and anxieties, to note perhaps too some prejudices and premises, but to enter each lecture as open-minded as you can be: Lecture equals opportunity, if I but let it. I may discover ways to indicate my anxieties without embarrassing myself before my peers. I might discover that the tutor shares a deep concern for patient experience that more than matches my own! I need to arrive on time, be mentally fresh and give myself to the discussion that happens there.

The above discussion considers mental preparation, students' attitudes towards lectures, and the importance of remaining receptive to alternative ideas that emerge there. But what of practical preparations for a lecture? What is important here? Make a list of those that occur to you.

Our suggestions are provided at the end of the chapter.

Engaging with the lecture

As we have seen in Table 4.1, lectures may take different forms and they are by no means always dry presentations. Tutors find imaginative ways to interact with students. For example, we have used multi-coloured cubes placed before each student in the lecture theatre, enabling the group as a whole to respond to periodic questions that we pose. We ask students to respond using the different coloured faces of their cubes. Each colour corresponds to an answer from a series of options that appear on the PowerPoint screen. In a lecture on healthcare policy implementation, we might ask the audience which of six options best describes who should be consulted on making the policy work. Perhaps some students show a red face (indicating the healthcare team) and others a yellow face (senior healthcare managers). We hope, though, that most will show the green face of the cube (healthcare teams, managers, patients and lay carers). The tutor is then able both to understand what the students think and to debate with them why particular choices have been made.

Engagement, however, is not limited to responding to tutors' questions. It involves attending to the lecture in different ways at different points. Successful students listen with a purpose. De Bono (2000), in a famous account of different ways of thinking, referred to six differently coloured hats that related to the nature of thinking that people might usefully engage in. Each of the metaphorical coloured hats described a different way of attending to what was being said.

- **White hat thinking** focuses upon the data, the facts and the figures. White hat thinking is concerned with evidence and involves the thinker in questions about what we already know. What is already clear in this data and what don't we yet know? White hat thinking is very important, for instance, when we consider statistics. What do experts think the incidence of hospital admissions linked to a pandemic infection might be?
- **Red hat thinking** is concerned with intuition, feelings, emotions and experience. Aspects of nursing care have the potential to evoke strong emotions within us and to reveal, through these, things about our values and beliefs. In a lecture on nursing ethics, where case studies are presented, you might need to attend to the feelings evoked.
- **Black hat thinking** describes a more cautious and judgemental form of thinking. It engages the thinker in a debate about whether arguments can be supported. It is not assumed that you will leave every lecture agreeing with the tutor. Indeed, in many instances the lecture will have served to highlight what your alternative account of matters might be and to prompt reflections on what evidence supports each view.
- **Yellow hat thinking** refers to logical reasoning and especially that which concerns whether something will work. You might use this sort of reasoning in association

with theories presented within the lecture. Can these be applied in practice and, if so, to what extent? If a theory–practice gap exists, how big is this and why does it arise?

- **Green hat thinking** is the sort that demonstrates your creativity. It involves you in proposing new ideas and suggestions. In a lecture, it might prove to be important when the tutor invites you to speculate about an ideal form of care delivery, or a better way to run a service.
- **Blue hat thinking** refers to what we have previously called metacognition, and engages you in a review of the process of what is going on here. In a lecture, it might be used to sit back and to reflect on the direction in which a debate about vaccination programmes is going. What are we in fact doing here, agreeing there?

While the structure and format of a lecture are limited only by the imagination of the tutor and the need to secure particular learning objectives, there are some classic features of most lectures to which we can apply the different thinking hats. In doing this you are a strategist, switching the way in which you think to suit the different features of the lecture that you come across. The better strategist you become, the more you will be able to integrate learning here to that which you do within other parts of your course; for example, asking questions about how clinical experiences and lecture messages mutually reinforce one another and give you the confidence to practise in a particular way.

Typically a lecture will include:

- **scene-setting and context-relating** – the tutor asks students to focus on a particular subject matter, often linked to lecture goals or objectives;
- **exposition** – where the tutor summarises points discovered through research, presented as theory or indicated by experience; exposition is typically happening when the tutor refers to the literature or states a particular theory;
- **illustration** – tutors sometimes draw on their own personal experience of nursing, or that shared by other practitioners;
- **speculation** – where the tutor debates issues, or different expositions; for example, two or more theories of counselling may have been shared and the tutor considers the relative merits of each;
- **interrogation and consultation** – where the tutor invites responses from students, either to check their understanding or to engage them further in the subject matter; dependent on the audience size there may be scope for limited group activity;
- **summation** – where the tutor sums up what the lecture has conveyed;
- **next direction** – where the tutor suggests what further work, reading or reflection is now useful.

Activity 4.3   *Critical thinking*

Look now at Table 4.2, where you will see a list of the ways of thinking described by de Bono (1985) and the classic features of a lecture. Decide which of the thinking hats might work best with each of the classic features of a lecture listed. You should be aware that, for some features of a lecture, more than one thinking hat may be applicable. Just which one you choose will be influenced by your past studies, current confidence regarding the subject of the lecture and your reactions to the way the tutor presents information.

Our solution is shared at the end of the chapter.

Table 4.2: Ways of attending to lecture content.

Features of the lecture	Possible thinking hats
1. Scene-setting and context-relating	a. White hat: focusing on the facts or figures (what do we know and what don't we know?)
2. Exposition	b. Red hat: intuition, feelings and emotions
3. Illustration	c. Black hat: caution and judgement
4. Speculation	d. Yellow hat: thinking about the practicalities
5. Interrogation and consultation	e. Green hat: creativity
6. Summation	f. Blue hat: stepping back; what is happening in this lecture, where are we going?
7. Next direction	

Listening and making notes

To think in the above ways, quizzically and reflectively, testing your own assumptions and those of others, is only possible if you are able to listen attentively. But many students report difficulties with this, as they explain that they are busily writing down information that the tutor has shared. Attending a lecture is seen as an information-gathering expedition and the student then erroneously believes that, because they have amassed a set of notes, they have learnt successfully. It is our experience that, in making extensive notes, there is little scope for the depth or the quality of thinking that helps students to master new subjects or to develop analytical ways of proceeding. A balance needs to be struck between making sufficient notes to aid memory and to prompt activities post-lecture (perhaps writing an assignment), and immersing yourself in the subject of the lecture, thinking carefully about what the tutor says.

There is a real advantage, then, in negotiating with your tutor to have the basic information associated with the lecture made available as a handout. If this comes in the form of a PowerPoint presentation, the slide summaries can be issued at the start of the lecture and students are able to annotate each with reflections that help capture the discussions that ensued. Where a tutor does not wish to reveal all of the information in the presentation at the start of a lecture, it is still possible for a handout to be provided at the end, or perhaps posted on a course website for students interested in the subject to download. The latter has the advantage that excess use of paper is reduced and annotated documents can then be added by the student, directly into their electronic portfolio of learning. What is important is that you establish at the start of the lecture what basic information will be made available by the tutor. If a handout is provided or downloadable, you are free to make briefer and more personally relevant notes regarding what you think as the lecture unfolds.

Activity 4.4 Critical thinking

Put your metaphorical black thinking hat on now and decide whether you support the above argument about intensive note-taking and the limitations that this sets on thinking in lectures. If you support our argument, consider how you will negotiate handout arrangements with your tutors. If you disagree, what is it about your note-taking that permits you to think deeply as you write?

We don't propose an answer to this activity because it serves simply to help you think about what works for you. We suggest, though, that in more complex and unfamiliar subjects, thinking time within the lecture is valuable.

The notes that you do make within a lecture should be sufficient to remind you what was said, in order to trigger later reflections and aid revision. It is unrealistic to write extensive notes at the pace that lectures proceed, and to try to do so will leave you frustrated at what you missed. Your notes, then, should be rather like those of a sports journalist who is reporting from a football match – representing events, but still allowing you to attend to the new things that you are seeing and hearing. Three of the techniques that you might use include the following.

- Simply list key words or short phrases that capture the essential features of the subject – so much the better if you add exclamation marks or question marks to remind you about what was surprising or seemed questionable. For these to work, you need to commit to 'writing up notes' as soon as possible after the lecture.
- A variant of this is to use a spider diagram, by placing the key concepts centre stage on a piece of paper and then adding branches of related ideas or points, using arrows to show what leads to what and what interacts with other things (see Figure 4.1).

Figure 4.1: Illustration of a spider diagram relating to part of a lecture on altered body image in cancer.

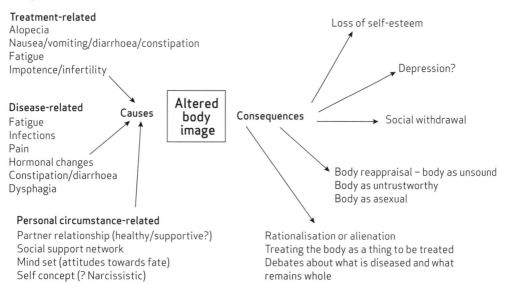

Treatment-related
Alopecia
Nausea/vomiting/diarrhoea/constipation
Fatigue
Impotence/infertility

Disease-related
Fatigue
Infections
Pain
Hormonal changes
Constipation/diarrhoea
Dysphagia

Personal circumstance-related
Partner relationship (healthy/supportive?)
Social support network
Mind set (attitudes towards fate)
Self concept (? Narcissistic)

Causes → **Altered body image** → Consequences

Loss of self-esteem
Depression?
Social withdrawal
Body reappraisal – body as unsound
Body as untrustworthy
Body as asexual

Rationalisation or alienation
Treating the body as a thing to be treated
Debates about what is diseased and what remains whole

- Summarise only that evidence, or this theory, that the discussion then proceeds from. You will recall the debates afterwards and can add some further points that emerge as you reflect on the lecture afterwards.

The use of questions to facilitate learning

Questions feature regularly within lectures, although many students worry about these. They fear that a question posed by the tutor will seem unanswerable and that, in not venturing an answer, or offering the wrong answer, their reputation will be blemished. They are concerned, too, that to ask questions of the tutor may also signal their ignorance, either because the question may seem naive to others, or because they fear that the tutor may rebuke their question as in some sense inappropriate. You will only develop your critical thinking abilities, however, if you are prepared to engage in questions, asking your own and answering those of your tutor or colleagues. Questions enable you to fill in gaps in your knowledge and to ascertain whether your current grasp of a subject is complete. Tutors know that it feels daunting for a student to engage in this, so they use a technique that allows the more confident students to venture answers to questions first. As you attend your next lecture, notice how the tutor poses a question first to the whole group, inviting possible answers from students. The tutor 'poses' the question, then 'pauses', allowing time for everyone to give the question due consideration, and then 'pounces'. Lest pounce sounds rather intimidating, remember that pose/pause/pounce is simply an aide-memoire for teachers learning their craft. The pounce usually involves inviting a student who has signalled interest in answering to proceed with their point. Tutors are taught *not* to embarrass individual students in the class. Where your answer is incomplete, you will usually be congratulated on the successful part of the answer before the tutor invites others to add to it. 'Gina has given us part of the answer here; who can add some more?'

Posing your own questions requires a little thought. It is important to configure a question that is comprehensible to the tutor – one that perhaps others too might wish to hear an answer on – and to ensure that this is a question and not a comment. Students frequently mix the two up, leaving the tutor unsure how best to respond, or at worst to feel that their teaching has been undermined. In the meantime, you may sound confused to your colleagues, or perhaps opinionated. Here is Stewart, posing a very successful question associated with the lecture on cancer and altered body image:

> *I was interested in the points that you made about the sort of cancer that patients have and the effect of this on their body image. Some tumours are especially threatening. I've recently nursed a man who had a mouth cancer and he has had to have radical surgery. I wondered whether cancers that affect the face are especially distressing?*

In this example, Stewart does three things. First, he orientates the tutor to where his question is focused: 'I was interested in the points that you made about . . .'. Second, he gives the briefest rationale for posing the question: 'I've recently nursed a man . . .'. Then he poses the question itself: 'I wondered whether . . .'. Stewart may already have a good idea that patients with head and neck cancers suffer a higher incidence of altered body image. He has witnessed their distress. But he still manages to phrase this as a question that the tutor can answer and others can understand. Had he wished to venture a tentative opinion, and had invited the tutor to either support or disagree with him, the question could have been posed differently:

I have just finished a placement on the head and neck cancer unit and colleagues there seem to deal with a lot of psychological distress in patients with oral, facial or neck cancers. I've played with the idea that this is because the face is so important for our personal identity and wondered whether you think that this is a supportable idea?

As you look at the above offerings from Stewart, you might usefully reflect that the first is the more traditional question. Here, Stewart doesn't expose so much of his own thinking and it is a good way forward if you feel less sure about the subject of the lecture. If you were feeling more confident, though, and wished to check your understanding, the second would be a reasonable and clear way to present the question.

Activity 4.5	Reflection

In the next lecture that you attend, give particular attention to the ways in which questions are posed by students – those that ask for an answer and those that help the individual to check the reasonableness of their ideas. Does the quality of questioning significantly enhance what you take away from a lecture? What do you think that the student who asks questions takes away from the session, that other students might not? Look back to your answer to Activity 4.1 and decide whether you wish to upgrade the part that questioning plays in a successful lecture.

As this activity is based on your own reflection, there is no answer at the end of the chapter.

After the lecture has finished

Irrespective of whether you did or didn't make extensive notes within a lecture, or whether you answered or ventured questions of your own, we would encourage you not to leave the lecture to one side after it has finished. If it is to make a coherent contribution to the rest of your studies, there are some things that you can do now that will not only reinforce your learning, but will help motivate your next enquiries as well. Here is our 'to do' list.

- Expand on your notes in order to produce a resource that can assist you with assessments that might lay special emphasis on the command of facts. You may need to consult a textbook to clarify your thinking at this point. Writing points out as paragraphs forces you to express your reasoning in ways that lists cannot.
- Identify any points of continuing interest – things that you either don't understand completely or that seem worth following up. Where will you find the new information? Perhaps this is something that will be available through a discussion in your personal tutor group. It may be something that a clinical placement mentor can help you with.
- Make a reflective note concerning your perceptions at this point. If you found some of the arguments made by the tutor unsettling or startling, determine why this is. What within your past experience, attitudes or values led you to alternative perspectives? What if anything needs to change now? Now is a good time to commit your reflections to your portfolio and to consider whether you need to discuss any insights that you may have with others.

C H A P T E R   S U M M A R Y

The lecture is probably the learning opportunity that students think they know the most about and sometimes get the least from. Over-exposure to lectures and making assumptions that one can get by simply by 'listening in' to the key points can undermine what can be achieved by full engagement with a lecture. Lectures are a common feature within nursing courses, so it is foolish not to derive the maximum benefit from them. By engaging with the lecture and its subject matter, you can not only learn a great deal, but you can contribute to the successful learning of others. This chapter has highlighted ways in which different sorts of thinking can relate to different features of the lecture, and how questions that you then pose as well as answer materially enrich everyone's learning.

Preparing carefully for the lecture and following up with reflective notes will significantly enhance what you learn. Materially, though, it is perhaps the quality of thinking within the lecture that determines whether you will develop the inquisitive attitudes that are so important in nursing. In the lecture, you witness the reasoning of another – the tutor. In the years that follow, opportunities to attend lectures, and to witness reasoning writ large, will be few. Learning to use such opportunities now will equip you to go on learning, within your current course and throughout your career.

Activities: brief outline answers and reflections

Activity 4.1: Reflection (page 52)

We thought that the following lecture was impressive. It was delivered at an international conference to an audience of 400 delegates, and concerned body image and the difficulties experienced by nurses as they tried to talk about this intimate subject with patients. The lecturer began with an exercise, inviting the delegates to stare at their neighbours for 30 seconds, noting the physical features of the other person. Next, the lecturer asked delegates to close their eyes and to imagine the other person's appearance once more. He asked a series of questions about the images delegates held in their minds. What was the colour of the other person's eyes? Were there any blemishes on their teeth? Were there any moles and, if so, could the delegate recall just where these appeared? After each question the delegates were invited to raise their hands if they felt sure they knew the answer. The lecturer reported the confidence rate: colour of eyes – 40 per cent thought they knew this; moles and teeth blemishes – 10 or perhaps 15 per cent affirmed a clear memory. He explained at the end of the exercise that the delegates had demonstrated how hard it was to recall the images of others and speculated with them that this was because they had been concerned at their own appearance being under scrutiny. To attend to another person's body image we need to be comfortable with our own. The audience laughed; relaxed with the difficult subject matter of the lecture. Their attention was gained and the end of the session produced a flood of interested and well-informed questions that everyone benefited from.

Activity 4.2: Critical thinking (page 54)

The preparations that we make vary depending on the lecture concerned. For example, if it is one of a series, it would be important to refer back to previous notes and handouts, because the tutor might well refer to themes begun there. Other very practical preparations include:

- reading any set texts notified by the tutor;
- completing any preliminary practical work (e.g., bringing some opening definitions along of the topic that would be discussed);
- noting how the lecture relates to course learning outcomes and assessments; some lectures may be pivotal to future assessed work;
- briefly indicating in note form what you think you do and don't know about this subject so far;
- posing one or two draft questions that you hope the lecture will assist you with; for example, do psychoses tend to change as the patient ages?

Activity 4.3: Critical thinking (page 55)

- **Scene setting** (blue hat). We think that, at the outset, you need to think quite hard about what this lecture will add to your understanding and to contemplate if there remain any gaps. Remember, your course of studies has been unique, and your clinical experiences different from those of others.
- **Exposition** (red, black and yellow hats). Exposition may be returned to at several points in the lecture by the tutor, so don't assume that features of the lecture appear in a linear fashion! Red hat thinking may be important though, as the lecture says something that challenges you. How will I respond to that – reject it, note it down, perhaps ask a private question at the end of the lecture? We might disagree with a tutor, but if our emotions then block out all else that is taught we are the loser. The black hat is important here too. Under what conditions is what the tutor says true, defensible, proven? Should we draw on clinical experience to debate such matters? We think the yellow hat comes into play because, if what the tutor says is true, we need to ask what the implications are of this. If holistic care involves a deep appreciation of spiritual and psychological well-being, social and physical needs, what are the implications when trying to deliver holistic care in a short-stay hospital ward?
- **Illustration** (yellow hat). We find that, when tutors illustrate points, we are prompted to think too about our experiences. Does their illustration help us understand our experience?
- **Speculation** (red, yellow and green hats). The lecturer's speculations tend to show how they frame a subject, to see it as a fact, problem or opportunity for instance. This may trigger old emotions, prompt cautions evaluation, imagine implications. We might say, 'goodness, I could think about this in a whole new way!'
- **Interrogation and consultation** (green and white hats). Asked a question, we necessarily search around for what we know, what counts as fact and what can be offered as the answer! But we might also try some creative thinking as we pose questions of our own. What if care was like this; do you think that would be better?
- **Summation** (yellow and black hats). As the tutor sums up the lecture, it is appropriate to consider to what extent we support the points he or she has made. We also debate what the implications of this might be, for our practice, our learning and the work that we still need to do.
- **Next direction** (green and blue hats). If the lecture has been inspiring, we may be motivated to study further and to ask new and creative questions about how we think and work. We go green. Our blue hat thinking concerns the fitting of this lecture to other learning that has been completed. What do I now understand as a result of a combination of these things?

Knowledge review

To help you determine what you have taken from this chapter, answer the following questions, making brief notes as seem appropriate in your portfolio.

1. In what ways do you now see lectures afresh? (Are they more or less of a resource than you anticipated?)
2. How can our assumptions prior to lectures affect learning in them?
3. Why do we need to think in different ways during the course of a lecture?
4. What are the features of a successful question?
5. Why is it important to write up notes after the lecture has ended?

Further reading

Browne, N and Keeley, S (2009) *Asking the Right Questions*, 9th edition. Boston, MA: Allyn & Bacon.
This book builds on what you have already read within this text on critical thinking and the importance of questions. It forms a good adjunct to the material that you have read on 'thinking hats'. While this and the other books recommended here don't focus on nursing or even healthcare, the concepts discussed have widespread application.

Buzan, T and Buzan, B (2006) *The Mind Map Book*. London: BBC Active.
For those of you who are interested in making spider diagrams or 'mind maps', this is an extremely valuable book and provides the arguments regarding why visual maps of ideas, as opposed to lists, are so powerful as aids to memory and reasoning.

de Bono, E (1985) *Six Thinking Hats*. New York: Little Brown.
This is an indulgence read, when you are not pressed for time and preparing for assessments! It is a book about thinking within the wider world of business and commerce, and about the ways in which teams work and corporations thrive. Consider, though, are these thinking hats equally important in healthcare teams and organisations? A visit to this classic reference is amply rewarded as you study nursing management.

Useful websites

www.open.ac.uk/skillsforstudy (Skills for OU Study)
The Open University has a long-established record of successfully helping students to study, and this includes guidance on note-taking, from what is heard and what is read. This comprehensive site includes wide-ranging practical tips on getting the most from your teaching, in whichever form it comes.

www.educationatlas.com
Study Skills Guide for Students, EducationAtlas.com
As well as acquainting students with a wide range of different university courses, this site offers a simple and accessible guide to study skills. The guidance is succinct and practical.

Chapter 5

Making sense of workshops

NMC Standards for Pre-registration Nursing Education (2010)

This chapter will address the following competencies.

Domain: Professional values

6. All nurses must understand the roles and responsibilities of other health and social care professionals, and seek to work with them collaboratively for the benefit of all who need care.

Domain: Communication and interpersonal skills

4. All nurses must . . . use effective communication strategies and negotiation techniques to achieve best outcomes, respecting the dignity and human rights of all concerned. They must know when to consult a third party and how to make referrals for advocacy, mediation or arbitration.

Domain: Leadership, management and team working

6. All nurses must work independently as well as in teams. They must be able to take the lead in coordinating, delegating and supervising care safely, managing risk and remaining accountable for the care given.
7. All nurses must work effectively across professional and agency boundaries, actively involving and respecting others' contributions to integrated person-centred care. They must know when and how to communicate with and refer to other professionals and agencies in order to respect the choices of service users and others, promoting shared decision making, to deliver positive outcomes and to coordinate smooth, effective transition within and between services and agencies.

Chapter aims

By the end of this chapter you will be able to:

*   define what is meant by workshop learning in its different forms;
*   compare and contrast the critical thinking required within lectures and workshops;

- make arguments about the benefits of workshop learning as part of a nurse's preparation for practice;
- reflect on what seems personally challenging and exciting about workshop learning;
- detail how the management of uncertainty and working towards clear workshop products can help to sustain study;
- explain why the working relationship with the tutor changes in workshop learning.

Introduction

Some of the most influential learning within your course of studies is likely to happen in one or other form of workshop. We use the term here to describe all facilitated learning activities, where some type of group interaction and peer-supported learning features as part of the plan. The oft-heard aphorism, 'what I see or hear I forget; what I do, I remember', is true in our experience. A workshop involves significant student participation and usually this is combined with a less directive, more facilitative role for the tutor (Lucas, 2009). Instead of teaching you the subject, the tutor aids your discovery of it. Learning is likely to be inductive (whereby you create explanations for what is experienced) and deductive (where you then take an emergent explanation and see if that fits with other contexts as well). It will often combine insights into skills and knowledge, and in ways that might be applied in practice, project working or team building. Among the workshops that you might be invited to take part in are the following.

- **Masterclasses**, where an expert practitioner helps you to rehearse your practice skills. Masterclasses combine demonstration with guidance and feedback as you attempt to emulate practice. Supportive feedback on your performance is encouraged from the rest of the study group. Example: listening techniques to assist anxious patients.
- **Problem-based learning sessions** (Price, 2003a), which are typically based on patient care scenarios and where you and your colleagues are invited to use available evidence to work out what the important issues are, what is problematic and how you will then proceed. Example: managing a patient's chronic pain.
- **Journal clubs**, where you collectively review one or more papers and then develop your critical faculties by discussing the content and the presentation of the article. Example: critical review of research design.
- **Action-learning sets** (Marsick and O'Neil, 2007), where you are asked to bring events and issues from your clinical practice to the group, with a view to collectively enhancing your understanding of nursing work. After each group meeting you take new questions back into clinical care, the better to understand the work that you do. Example: change agency skills of the nurse leader.
- **Fact-finding projects**, where the group members are each tasked with the search for important information, and the collectively secured information is then used to provide a new account of nursing care. Facts may be found in the library, the media, within clinical practice or through interviews of others. Example: policies and strategies to deal with influenza pandemics.
- **Online exercises**, which may again be about problem solving, but equally importantly are to acquaint you with technology and allow you to debate points

with peers in a mutual and virtual reality. Example: exploring international perspectives on the role of the nurse.

This is a just a selection. Your teachers may have other ideas.

Workshops are important in nursing curricula because, as a healthcare professional, you will later be charged with finding out your own information, determining where and how to search for evidence, and collaborating with colleagues to achieve goals. If your studies solely consisted of lectures and clinical practice, it would be much more difficult for you to develop a more independent and collegiate form of learning. Workshops, then, are not as one student once suggested a means for the tutor to gain some respite from teaching. They are carefully structured activities that require the tutor to operate in a less directive way. Your tutor will step in where work is coming off the track, but will not direct your thinking, discussion, decisions and future plans moment by moment.

In this chapter we summarise what is different about workshop forms of learning and explore what is most challenging and exciting in connection with these. We make the case that, while you may favour a more passive and private form of learning, you will develop both your critical thinking and your reflective practice skills if you engage wholeheartedly in such sessions. Some of the things that facilitate learning are under the tutor's control, while others are under your control. Good workshop design is the work of the tutor. Working with others to manage uncertainty within the workshop group is yours. You will need to set aside the notion that colleagues cannot teach you as well as the tutor, and examine what collective experience offers. We suggest that working towards a discernible product at the end of your workshop helps bring purpose to your work.

Activity 5.1   *Reflection*

Take a moment to reflect on any workshops that you have been involved in, and to determine whether they seemed successful.

- What did it feel like to learn together as a group?
- If the workshops were successful, what made them so?
- If they seemed wanting in some regard, what seemed to undermine them?

As this activity is based on your own reflection, there is no answer at the end of the chapter.

Where students typically report problems with workshop learning, it is usually because of one or more of three things. First, the learning seemed more arduous and less time-efficient than if a conventional lecture had been used. Students wondered what had been achieved there that could not have been done so using another learning method. A lack of insight into the purpose of workshops thwarted progress. Second, one or more people within the learning group undermined the project work being completed. Colleagues may have baulked at the work required and not contributed a fair share of effort. Third, the project seemed poorly structured and managed. Colleagues felt that they were left for too long to wonder and debate about an issue, when the group suspected that the tutor knew the answers anyway and could have been rather more supportive.

In our experience, where students report successful workshop learning, this is also typically associated with three things. First, there was a sense of achievement linked to the discoveries made, both those that were personal and those that the group managed between them. Second, there was surprise at what was discovered through group work, not merely about the subject of investigation, but about the process of working as a team. Colleagues in these groups noted that the learning was about processes as well as knowledge bases. Third, there was pleasure in working with others, within a group that seemed to 'gel'. Students reported that the purposeful association with others was stimulating and often reassuring in a field of practice that so often seemed to test the individual rather than recognise the work of the group.

In part, then, the success of a workshop is determined by your expectations of learning and their fit (or otherwise) with the requirements of the course. If your learning style is more private, perhaps more passive, and you are receptive and contemplative, rather than strategic and collaborative, workshop learning will seem more difficult. If you are inquisitive and explorative by nature, and enjoy working with others to achieve goals, workshop learning will seem attractive. However, nursing does emphasise team work and collaboration, and learning from experience, so workshops are an important way of learning (see, for example, Speck, 2006; McCray, 2009).

Managing uncertainty

At the heart of all workshop learning is the need to manage uncertainty. What is required of us, of me, and what shall we do to manage the project set before us? What might be achieved, missed, or perhaps misunderstood? What mistakes might happen to confuse our understanding of a subject or perhaps risk a loss of personal reputation, as a student and as a nurse? What might excite and motivate me for the future? If we can manage uncertainty, learning becomes more purposeful and pleasurable.

If, however, the workshop was designed to leave no questions remaining, no enquiries to conduct, and no issues to debate, there would be no scope for learning through experience. We would not understand what effort it takes to reach decisions, or to make policies or protocols, and we would not understand how groups can operate together to develop strategies of their own. Raymet felt the uncertainty of her group learning activities acutely. She recorded in her portfolio:

What alarmed me about the exercises was not only just how much we didn't know. No, what alarmed me was how little there was in this area that offered a right answer, the correct way to act. I craved assurance and only gradually learned to trust my team mates and myself, to make good decisions.

Activity 5.2   *Critical thinking*

Look now at the following list of possible ways to resolve group learning uncertainty and decide which of these could have helped you with past problems encountered while working with others. Don't worry if that experience comes from a past course or outside nursing, as the principles still hold good. As you examine these options, reflect on the extent to which each adds clarity of purpose to group working.

- Asking the tutor to clarify the project brief before you set off.
- Checking what arrangements are in place for ensuring that work proceeds in the right direction.

Activity 5.2 continued   *Critical thinking*

- Ascertaining what the aptitudes of group members are; for example, one colleague might be good at searching library databases.
- Setting out a schedule of work, agreeing what sorts of activity are needed and deciding in what order these will be tackled.
- Agreeing a means of recording your progress, the decisions that you have made and the discoveries made.
- Determining group etiquette, that is, an agreed way of talking about each other and colleagues' contributions.

We offer our reflections at the end of the chapter.

To complete your group activities, it is necessary to start with the clearest possible brief. If yours seems unclear, you should ask the tutor to clarify points for you. In most instances, group activities are supported by a written brief and starter materials. Within a problem-based learning exercise, for example, there is likely to be one or more patient case study and associated tasks to complete. Typically, too, the project will set out the aims and objectives of the exercise, so that you can sense what work is necessary.

While tutors don't direct the work of the group, they are required to keep a watching brief. To leave less experienced nurses without a source of guidance would be both unproductive and demotivating. It is a good idea, then, to check with the tutor when he or she will intervene to ensure that enquiries continue in an appropriate way. Consulting with the tutor on a regular basis in projects that span several weeks is important. Such 'check points' allow you to ascertain whether work is proceeding towards the required objectives, although your tutor is unlikely to give you a whole 'teaching staff solution'. Here is a typical response that Raymet received on a problem-based learning exercise:

I think that you're making good progress. The things that you are debating about epilepsy and social stereotypes are exactly what I would think about. But you need, too, to think about what propels the care plan forward. If worries paralyse you as well as the parents of this child, you won't be serving them very well. Have a think this week about what is known about managing epilepsy.

Project groups are usually composed of students with a mix of aptitudes, and it certainly isn't expected that all group members will be good at everything. Indeed, sometimes the tutor devises project groups to help students to explore and share their aptitudes. To gain the benefit of individual aptitudes, however, you will need to be prepared to volunteer what you feel comfortable doing, even if you believe that your work might not be perfect. You will need to acknowledge, too, the work done by others who have other talents. Setting aside personal insecurities is part of the learning process. Start with the assumption that we all have insecurities, many of which are unspoken. What is more important now is that what you share works to achieve project ends. Here is Raymet again:

I'm not imaginative or creative. I could see that Annette and Sean were the creative ones and that was so good. I thought to myself, you must work at this, you cannot rely on just these two. That was why I volunteered to make the notes and to sum up our decisions at different points. I was the scribe of our group and later on that was valuable, as we found so much information it would have been easy to have lost our way.

Wasted time increases the pressures on a group, especially as they near the point where they must present their findings. For that reason, agreeing a schedule of work and how much time is allocated to each part of the project helps to discipline the enquiry. Instead of a project that finishes with a lot of information about just one thing, you will have a project that seems balanced and measured, professional and insightful. As we have seen above, it is then necessary to keep a brief record of the lines of enquiry and the decisions made. Such an 'audit trail' enables the group to tell the story of their enquiry, as well as to present the end product of what they have learned. What did we consider, what did we conclude, what was left to one side for now and how did we arrive at our decisions?

Simple group etiquette rules ensure that colleagues are treated with respect and that each contributes in an adequate measure to the work in hand. For example, rules might set out expectations regarding attending meetings, supplying copies of interesting evidence found, and listening attentively until a colleague has presented the whole of their findings. Most project briefs will refer to such group etiquette and either set some parameters for you to follow or suggest which ones need to be agreed.

Creating an end product

Workshop activity prompts you to combine the skills of critical thinking and reflection that have been presented in Part 1 of this book. Because projects change over time, there is a need for reflection. Because projects demand of you decisions and selective use of resources, you have to think critically, discriminating what is worthy of your attention. Project work, however, is not open-ended and there is a need to reach closure, sharing what you have discovered with others and evaluating what the activity has taught you. It is to this end, to reach a closure that is satisfying and helpful, that nursing courses usually require some sort of 'end product' at the conclusion of the project.

Activity 5.3	Decision making

Consider now in Table 5.1 the different 'end products' that might be associated with workshop learning. We have paired these with different sorts of workshops in which they often appear. The associations are indicative, however; courses differ in what is required. In some instances, study groups have the opportunity to determine their own end products, especially if their projects have run over several weeks.

Next, refer back to Chapter 1 of this book and the discussion of critical thinking aptitudes. How do you think these project end products might assist you to develop the critical thinking aptitudes you have read about? Do some of these end products seem to you more comfortable or doable than others? If so, what does this tell you about your critical thinking development so far?

Make a note of your answers before referring to our thoughts at the end of the chapter.

Table 5.1: Workshop contexts and typical 'end products'.

Workshop context	Typical end products
Masterclass	A revised demonstration of a skill (e.g., using a manikin simulator, two video records are made of wound-dressing techniques, one before and one after the masterclass; you then invite the audience to make notes comparing the two performances)
Problem-based learning session	An illustrated verbal presentation to the wider group (in some instances more than one group explore the same problem, the better afterwards for everyone to discuss aspects of problem analysis) (e.g., working with families to manage childhood epilepsy)
Journal club	A collaborative, written critique of the chosen papers; the journal papers and their relevant critiques might then be made available through the library for wider consultation and discussion (e.g., a critique of papers that illustrate phenomenological research in nursing; comparisons and conclusions)
Action-learning set	A written guide on enhancing a named skill (this might be prepared as a teaching aide for more junior students) (e.g., psychological support for patients dealing with type 2 diabetes mellitus)
Fact-finding project	Both illustrated verbal and written reports are possible here, as are posters that might be presented at a study day or conference (e.g., a public health poster describing the ways in which influenza viruses are spread and what personal/public health measures may be used to counter the risk)
Online exercise	A written paper summarising discussions shared online and available for all to download (e.g., comparisons of nurses' roles, cultures and philosophies from four countries)

Working towards the workshop end product also contributes to your reflective abilities. While workshop activity linked to a long-term project has the greatest potential in this regard, all workshops have the potential to support some reflection. Figure 2.1 in Chapter 2 detailed the several benefits of reflection and we see a number of the above end products making a contribution here. For example, the written summary of nursing roles as understood in different countries and cultures, secured through online discussion with other student nurses at colleges abroad, could certainly teach us a great deal about the profession. In many regards, nursing is culturally defined (Burnard and Gill, 2008). What nurses deliver is determined in part by the society that they work in, especially with regard to lay carer and professional carer duties. This is a significant reflection when you work within a multicultural healthcare system.

Problem-based learning and fact-finding end products are likely to have helped to challenge your assumptions. It can be surprising to discover how often we rely on common-sense interpretations of situations. Discovering the facts and appreciating other ways to evaluate matters can prove revelatory. More generically still, and perhaps most importantly of all, group work teaches us about ourselves and others. What did you notice about ways of speaking, thinking and working together that helped to sustain the group through difficult times? What did you observe about the ways in which challenges were addressed? Are there lessons here that can later be transferred to clinical practice and the different initiatives that will be demanded of you and colleagues there?

Making best use of the tutor

One of the more profound changes that happen within workshops concerns the relationship between students and tutors. Tutors are eager to facilitate learning, rather than instruct. While some professional standards, etiquette and risk management points must be inculcated, much else that will sustain nurses after they have left the course will be achieved through a facilitation of enquiry. Strange as it can sometimes seem, your tutors work to render themselves redundant. They work to enable you to think, reflect and continue learning independently.

This prompts some reflections on the nature of communication between you and your tutors. We have noted the following.

- Tutors take a backward step and present ideas in much more tentative terms. While they don't wish to seem 'esoteric' about learning, they do try to prompt speculation.
- Tutors ask to be consulted on options and different explanations, rather than to confirm solutions. For example, you might debate with your tutor the relative merits of different ways of administering analgesia.
- Tutors sometimes gently provoke you, questioning your explanations of things. You need to recognise this for what it is – a challenge to think again, differently or more diversely.
- Students start to reappraise the skills and the reputation of their tutors. Do you need someone who is the fount of all knowledge – a 'book on legs' – or someone who helps you to think boldly? The tutor you sought and perhaps needed at the start of your course might be different from the one you seek and admire later on.

Activity 5.4   *Communication and team working*

Debate with colleagues the following assertion:

> *Workshop learning requires a form of emotional work; we need to pass through periods of uncertainty and difficulty in order to secure the best knowledge and insights. If tutors acted in a more directive way, we would never develop the skills we require.*

Formulate a case for this assertion and then some arguments against. How does this affect the way that you work with tutors in workshops? Have you begun to see your tutors' contributions in a new way?

We share brief reflections of our own at the end of the chapter.

CHAPTER SUMMARY

Learning with others does require an additional emotional effort, a significant degree of trust and some personal as well as collective organisation. It is certainly much easier to attend a lecture. The rewards of collaborating on workshop activities and longer-term projects, however, are considerable. There is a chance to pool experience, to draw on one another's critical thinking aptitudes and to develop the confidence needed to make decisions when a clear 'right answer' is not available. In many regards, the learning involved in workshops mimics that which happens within practice itself. We have to manage uncertainty and provide a structure for what we will do together. That means working towards end products and, whether this is the recovery of a patient or the completion of a project report, the clearer we are about these things the better.

Learning through workshops, though, does not preclude tutor involvement. Indeed, the measured contributions of the tutor are important, especially as students undertake their first workshop learning sessions. It is not enough for tutors to leave students to simply 'fly off and find out' (FOFO). What changes are the ways in which you enquire of the tutor. Instead of asking them to deliver the right answer, to assure and sustain, you ask them to share wise counsel. The tutor becomes the consultant of the group and you access their rehearsals of the merits and limitations of each point that you share: Yes, it could be that, but have you also considered . . .?

Because workshop activities necessarily expose you to uncertainty, you learn to manage the insecurity that attends it. You do so by working with peers, the self-same colleagues who will practise alongside you when you graduate. You combine critical thinking and reflection in ways that are unavailable to you in other forms of learning.

Activities: brief outline answers and reflections

Activity 5.2: Critical thinking (page 67)

All of these measures are extremely useful in giving a clarity and purpose to workshop learning. Each adds something to the structure of learning and helps you to attend in a more conscious, more strategic way. You might suppose, however, that workshop learning is flawed and this is because, as students, you don't know what you don't know! Surely it is the case that we cannot discover together that which none of us can conceive of or has experienced? Such a critique would be true but for three things. First, good workshops are designed to provide sufficient information and guidance based on what you have already been taught. They use information that the tutor knows you already have. Second, the chances of the whole group not having relevant knowledge or experience decreases as you progress through your course. Diverse clinical learning placements and student backgrounds mean that workshop groups can call upon a wider range of experience than you might anticipate. Third, the tutor stands ready to help you practise your speculation. In clinical practice, nurses don't know what they don't know about many problems presented to them. There will always be a patient who presents with the most unusual of circumstances. We come to understand, though, that working with bits of information that we do know and understand, and speculating what this might tell us about the rest, we can still proceed. We learn how to investigate.

Activity 5.3: Decision making (page 68)

Revised skill demonstration

You might note just how uncomfortable this learning could seem, but within a supportive group we think that this end product would certainly involve your ability to discriminate between good and not so good wound dressing in action, and to make selective arguments about how best to judge wound dressing skills. The healthcare world demands of nurses a series of competencies – those that support registered practice and those that underpin claims to advanced practice. Being able to explain what counts as competent and excellent is important.

A problem-based learning presentation

We think that the aptitudes of asking questions, discriminating, interpreting, speculating and making arguments are all at play here. Problem-based learning mimics the circumstances of nursing practice – a place where these aptitudes have to combine. The fact that two workshop groups provide different interpretations of the problem provides scope for further discussion.

A journal article critique

Journal article critiques are referenced against standards, for example those of validity, reliability and authenticity in research. So, as you critique the article, you will be making comparisons against the standards accepted. You will show discrimination and then make arguments about the merits of the paper.

Action-learning set report or other product

This sort of workshop activity seems to foster a great deal of interpretation and speculation. Each group member does this with regard to their own practice before the group asks a series of questions about what represents better practice. Because of the diversity of practice contexts and the complexity of work there, members may venture a number of different arguments about improving nursing care. Instead of a 'best way' to proceed, there may be 'best ways', each context-specific.

A poster (fact-finding project outcome)

Posters only have so much space for information, so you need to discriminate what will be included. What is it essential to explain here? A successful poster makes unambiguous arguments!

Online discussion written report

We thought that interpreting and speculating would be important here, acknowledging the cultural influences upon nursing. After that, there would be a series of questions asked – what do nurses share? Arguments might then be made to suggest that these are the things that characterise nursing internationally.

Activity 5.4: Communication and team working (page 70)

The extent to which you supported this statement is likely to be strongly related to your level of confidence as a learner and the point that you are at within your course of studies. Students approaching the end of a programme should (we believe) support an assertion such as this. Yes, learning involves emotional work, taking risks and dealing with uncertainty, but this is necessary and worthwhile. As learning progresses, the relationship with the tutor becomes more consultative and this is as we should expect. If you find near the end of your course that you strongly contest this assertion, it is worth discussing the matter with a personal tutor. What are the expectations here and why do your expectations seem out of sync with what we think examiners will expect?

Knowledge review

To help you check your grasp of the content of this chapter, answer the following questions. Relate your answers to your own personal experience and preferences regarding workshop learning.

1. What differentiates learning in a workshop from learning in a lecture?
2. State four things that are important and enable you to get involved fully with workshop learning. Write a short paragraph about each.
3. State four different forms of workshop learning and give examples of any that you have engaged in.
4. Critical thinking is changed in workshop learning and expressed in the different ways in which you consult the tutor. In one short paragraph, sum up that change.

Further reading

Azer, S (2008) *Navigating Problem Based Learning.* Edinburgh: Churchill Livingstone. This is a useful guide for any nurse engaged in studies that follow the principles of problem-based learning. It covers the part played by the tutor, by material prompts, and the nature of work then conducted by students as they make sense of available information.

Pedler, M (2008) *Action Learning for Managers.* Aldershot: Gower.
Action-learning sets are commonly associated with postgraduate nursing studies, but the principles are applied within a wide variety of courses. If you want to learn more about action learning, this is a helpful guide that describes the many features of the approach. Don't be put off if you are not yet a manager – the principles still apply.

Thompson, N (2009) *People Skills.* Basingstoke: Palgrave Macmillan.
What Neil Thompson has to teach about interpersonal skills is relevant across the healthcare services, but is especially important in workshop learning and small group projects. If you are intrigued by the process of project group work, or have encountered interpersonal problems there, this is a good book to dip into.

Useful websites

Rather than recommend specific websites on this occasion, we commend a search of the internet using the search term 'healthcare workshops'. This reveals the diverse ways in which workshops are conceived and run, and will serve to help tutors diversify their course curriculum. For students, it highlights what is possible within workshop learning, some of which remains available beyond graduation.

Chapter 6

Making sense of clinical placements

NMC Standards for Pre-registration Nursing Education (2010)

This chapter will address the following competencies.

Domain: Professional values

1. All nurses must practise confidently according to *The Code: Standards of conduct, performance and ethics for nurses and midwives* (NMC, 2008), and within other recognised ethical and legal frameworks. They must be able to recognise and address ethical challenges relating to people's choices and decision-making about their care, and act within the law to help them and their families and carers find acceptable solutions.
8. All nurses must practise independently, recognising the limits of their competence and knowledge. They must reflect on these limits and seek advice from, or refer to, other professionals where necessary.

Domain: Communication and interpersonal skills

1. All nurses must build partnerships and therapeutic relationships through safe, effective and non-discriminatory communication. They must take account of individual differences, capabilities and needs.
2. All nurses must use a range of communication skills and technologies to support person-centred care and enhance quality and safety. They must ensure people receive all the information they need in a language and manner that allows them to make informed choices and share decision making.

Chapter aims

By the end of this chapter you will be able to:

- summarise the nature of critical enquiry that you need to engage in within clinical placements;
- detail what preparations will enable you to complete a successful clinical placement;
- discuss the part played by the student–mentor relationship in a satisfying and effective learning placement;

- understand the reflective and open approach that you must use if mentor and other feedback is to aid your studies;
- appraise what it takes to work successfully with continuous assessment of learning in clinical placements.

Introduction

You are about to venture forth on your first clinical placement. What will it be like? What are the expectations associated with the placement? Will you make mistakes and can the staff tolerate that? Will there be someone there to support you? Irrespective of whether you are now a veteran of many such clinical placements or approaching your first one, the above questions and ones like them are likely to sound familiar. Learning within the clinical setting is exciting but potentially stressful, and it is helpful to understand why that is, and what you can do to counter the anxieties.

In this chapter, we explain what is different about learning in the clinical setting, what you should do when preparing to join a clinical placement, how you might work better with your mentor there, and what might be done to ensure that you do well in clinically based assessments. We will pay particular attention to the skills of observation, questioning, interpreting and speculating as they apply there. Critical thinking and reflection have a particular resonance here, because of the wealth and diversity of information that you will encounter. These skills will play a central role in helping you to both enjoy and learn from the time you spend in the clinical area.

Why clinical learning is different

We asked Gina to make four key points about why clinical learning was different. Here are the observations that she made:

What immediately impressed me was that this was a workplace and that learning had to be much more 'on the hoof'. That shouldn't have surprised me, but honestly, the impact of this change is bigger than you imagine. You forget how centre stage you are in the classroom, how much your learning means to the teaching staff. The clinical staff care, but learning has to fit in with the delivery of services.

The second thing I noted was that some of their teaching wasn't about the skill of nursing, it was about the etiquette of practice. I was being socialised into the team and being taught about where, how and when to ask questions. On reflection, that wasn't surprising as clinical practice is a theatre, it's where the public witness what we do. The staff were anxious about whether I might damage their reputation.

The third thing I noticed was how difficult it was to obtain a rationale for what was being done. You suddenly realise how much trained staff carry in their heads. I felt like a child, always wanting someone to answer the question 'why'! Clearly, the nurses couldn't always answer those questions, and especially in front of anxious patients. You had to wait for explanations.

The fourth thing I would say is that you face an information deluge. By that I mean you cannot stop to consider all the options, not as you might wish to anyway. It was the speed of thinking that blew me away and made me wonder whether I would ever learn here.

Gina offers an excellent summary of what makes learning in the clinical environment different. There is far less structure to the learning experience, certainly when compared to a well-run lecture. Students are required to seize the initiative and ask pertinent questions about what is happening. Certainly, clinical mentors are mindful not to overestimate students' confidence or ability, but they don't automatically remember to explain points that to them are second nature. There is, then, a need to choose when to ask the right questions, and Gina makes a good point when she infers that questions can seem impertinent if asked at the wrong moment. Learning the etiquette of enquiry is important, not only because it helps you to become part of the clinical team, but also because it enables the practitioners to carry on their work.

What Gina's account emphasises is the need to think in an inductive way: 'What is happening here?' Such questions are designed to help you make sense of a flood of experiences, and this is highlighted by Gina as she talks about the speed at which colleagues think. Clinical placements can overload you with information, and it isn't presented in a coherent form (Stuart, 2007). You are presented with a series of jigsaw pieces that you will need to fit together to create a picture. Some of those pieces you already have; they come from your past lectures, the theory of nursing and lessons on physiology, pharmacology and practical skills. Others will become available in placement – those connected with the patients, their diagnoses and current treatments. This situation reflects the reality of practice for qualified staff as well. All must continue to make sense of events, and the challenges and needs that arise wherever patients are cared for.

So, to learn effectively in clinical placements you will need to be inquisitive, sensitive to others around you (judging the right time to ask), analytical as you piece together disparate pieces of information, and diligent (trying to summarise what you have learned at the end of each shift) (Kassirer et al., 2009). You will need to deal with a greater level of uncertainty than you may have previously been accustomed to, but you are also likely to be reassured as more experienced nurses describe their own learning curve. As one nurse advised Gina:

One of the things you learn here is how to reason, how to build up a picture of what is required by a patient. You learn to accept that you are always learning, always questioning your last ideas. You don't do that on your own; the team help you and expect you to share what you think as the process continues.

So, to Gina's list of characteristics of clinical learning, we would add a fifth important point, and this is that learning here is communal. Elsewhere you may have learned in a more private and personal way. In the clinical area there is less scope for private deliberation. The team only learns how best to care for patients if its members share their incremental insights. This is ably illustrated in a number of processes that you will witness, including:

- 'teaching' rounds, where clinicians deliberate on care strategies;
- report handovers, where the team deliberate on the care delivered so far and where new priorities are identified;
- case conferences, where individual patient care is discussed in some depth and next steps are contemplated.

Look back now to Gina's four points regarding what makes clinical learning different, and draw upon any personal experience gained so far to illustrate these in action. For example, can you cite examples of where you think you were being socialised into the clinical team? Before leaving this activity, decide whether you can cite any further examples of clinical processes that emphasise the communal nature of learning in the clinical setting.

At the end of the chapter we offer observations concerning difficulties that some students have had to overcome as they shifted from college to clinical learning environments.

Preparing for the placement

Preparation for your placement can significantly reduce the anxiety that you feel on your first days there. The more you can bring structure and order to the learning experience, working with your mentor, the more constructive the learning will seem. Table 6.1 suggests what might be done in advance of your placement.

Table 6.1: Getting ready for clinical placement study.

Strategy	Benefit
Review the learning outcomes that have to be achieved during this placement and any assessment arrangements that apply.	You focus on what has to be achieved.
Research the work of the department, ward or practice by looking at any details on hospital websites and by asking students who have had placements there before.	By asking some preliminary questions you won't have to ask quite so many on your placement. Interpreting what is going on will seem easier.
Revisit your portfolio to identify particular practice skills that you wish to improve on, for example patient history taking.	You calmly discriminate what needs your attention. Explaining where you would like particular guidance helps the mentor to plan their support.
Make personal contact with the clinical team, writing or emailing the nurse in charge.	You establish an immediate rapport if you show such personal organisation. You make your first argument: I am diligent and well prepared and I value this placement.
Try to establish in advance who your mentor will be.	Knowing this, and whether you might share the same shift, will increase your confidence and is one less thing to think about later. Successful mentors' reputations sometimes go before them.

Check when your first shift is and arrive in good time, correctly attired.

Refer to your portfolio now and check whether there are practice skills that you promised to focus on in your next clinical placement. If not, write down in your portfolio three skills that you wish to develop further, adding a short rationale to each. Referring to these skills in your first conversation with your mentor will demonstrate your commitment and personal organisation. You are likely to get more from your mentor if you prove ready to seek information as well as to request it.

As this activity is based on your own reflection, there is no answer at the end of the chapter.

Observing, questioning, interpreting and speculating

Earlier, we referred to the importance of questioning within clinical placements and noted that questions often have to be reserved until later. It is worth anticipating what that will feel like now, so that you can ask questions more strategically when you are in the placement. Figure 6.1 outlines what typically happens.

1. Observations and experience

Learning starts with experience and clinical placements provide a constant stream of this. It is difficult to decide what to focus on, to consciously observe and to think about and what to let slip by. You cannot observe everything, neither can you analyse the whole experience before you. It is normal that you process only a percentage of the information available. Your observation will become more purposeful if you do four things.

- Note what seems most important to the patient. This usually means reading first and foremost what could entail risk for them and, after that, the events that may determine their experience of the quality of care. For example, the patient reports that they are allergic to penicillin. This needs noting down and reporting to others.
- Remember the learning outcomes that you need to achieve and the skills you wish to develop. It may help if you distil these into four or five priority interests. Lengthy lists of learning objectives are difficult to remember in the clinical area.
- Look for patterns of behaviour, and sequences of events that seem to tell a story about the nature of nursing care. For example, patient admission to hospital is a storyline and one that involves several nursing skills.
- Relate those observations that interest you most to your previous teaching. Does this confirm what you learned in class? Does it modify your understanding or augment the information that you received there?

2. Questions and emotions

Two things happen simultaneously at this point. You will certainly experience a number of emotions associated with what you experience in practice. You might note excitement, admiration, encouragement, confusion, disappointment, cynicism or anxiety. Experience is 'in the raw' here and you are confronted with an insight into nursing that may or may not support your preconceptions. The goal here, then, is to acknowledge honest feelings, but not to have them derail your learning. If you worry about, wonder at or even disapprove of

Figure 6.1: Learning in the clinical setting.

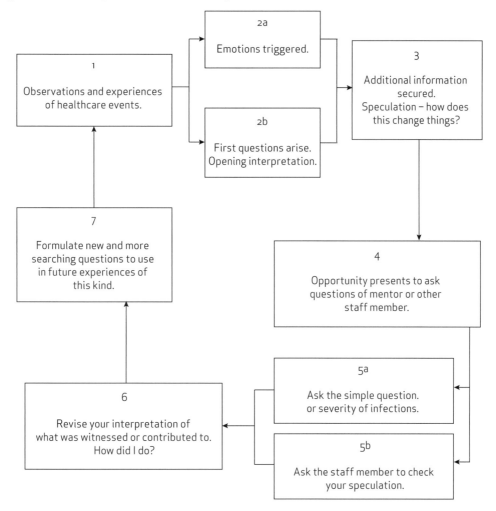

something witnessed, allow for a moment that you might not yet have all the information to allow a full evaluation. Mentally save those feelings and formulate a question about them for later. For example, 'I noted that you were very firm with Mrs Jones's daughter this morning. She had been warned that her mother would be discharged this week. Does that approach work best?'

Alongside the first emotions will be some questions in your mind and some initial interpretations of what is going on. These will constitute your first ideas about what is happening. In the above example, you may have wondered, 'could the nurse have seemed more empathetic towards this relative?' or 'what is at stake here, rehabilitating the patient, freeing up a much needed bed or expecting of a relative a shared duty of care?' If you are alert you will begin a tentative interpretation of the event. 'I suspect that this nurse has few choices. The need to attend to lots of patients places some limits on the extent to which she can personalise care.'

3. Additional information

It is highly likely that the stream of new information will continue coming your way. You need then to store your first thoughts and allow a new layer of thinking to develop. You are in the business of speculating. At this stage there is no guarantee that your ideas are correct, but speculation is still required. So, in our example, we may learn from the ward secretary that Mrs Jones's daughter works full time and that she has already lodged a request that her mother be held in hospital until the weekend. She was aware of the planned discharge, but hoped to argue that she could support her mother better if she was available during her first days at home. The additional information probably demonstrates the daughter's concern to be an active carer, but leaves doubts too about whether she trusts the other community care arrangements that have been put in place. You find yourself speculating further about systems and service, and about professional and lay care liaison. The nurse needs to work with a system, but advocate, where possible, the concerns of lay carers too.

4. Question opportunity

Opportunities to question arise later and in a variety of guises. It may be a one-to-one chat with the staff nurse during a coffee break, or opportunity for expression of concerns during a shift change. Nurses, doctors and others might invite questions after a ward round. The majority of such opportunities will be managed away from the audience of patients and lay carers. As we see below, there are two sorts of questions that could be asked, but irrespective of which you choose, it is necessary to demonstrate a respect for colleagues.

5. Asking your questions

Sometimes the complexity of things observed makes it difficult for you to pose anything other than a very simple question. 'What was problematic about the situation with Mrs Jones's daughter? I sensed a tension there.' Better by far, though, and with a trusted mentor, is to pose a question that invites them to check out your early speculation about events. 'I noticed the difficulty with Mrs Jones's daughter and started mulling over what that might be. I sensed that she wanted the discharge to work with her own arrangements; that she was really motivated to help with the transition home. But then again, she might have also been distrustful of the arrangements that we have made too. It isn't easy to find the compromise and we have to live with the discomforts of that . . . is that how you read it?'

6. Revising your interpretation

The answer you gain to your questions allow you to revise your interpretation of events. The interpretations may develop in several interesting ways and it is from this point that you can make some useful portfolio notes. For example, you might reinterpret your skill at reading practice episodes. Do I seem to be improving? You might re-examine your understanding of the mechanisms of hospital discharge and return to relevant policies.

Forming new questions

Having summed up your thoughts in the light of feedback, you are ready to observe practice with new insights. In our working example, you might consider in more detail how clinical colleagues work incrementally towards hospital discharge of a patient. How soon do they start preparing patients and carers for this? Do they always hear/ understand what others are saying? In the end, are there economic and logistic tensions that inherently underlie such things?

Study Figure 6.1 and consider whether the process of steps described there might assist you to be a more strategic learner in clinical practice. Why is it important to attend to what each step teaches us during the course of a placement?

We offer suggestions at the end of the chapter.

Working with your mentor

Students aren't always aware what a mentor brings to clinical supervision, so let us start with that. Mentors are experienced practitioners, who are familiar with their area of care and its local policies and protocols, who have undertaken a short course in the principles of learning, teaching, support and assessment, and who are charged with guiding you during your clinical placement. They act as advocates of learning, but they also have responsibilities to inculcate you into the team and its work. They work assiduously to help you to master necessary skills and apply your knowledge, but retain responsibilities towards their patients, colleagues and the profession. Mentors share unique insights into practice wisdom – the practical ways of conducting nursing work (Kinnell and Hughes, 2010).

Successful work with your mentor will:

- help you to manage your anxieties about learning in the clinical setting;
- help you to develop an acceptable approach to enquiry in this setting;
- open doors to other expertise in the clinical setting (a mentor might introduce you to colleagues with specialist knowledge and highlight your enthusiasm as a student);
- give you thoughtful and honest weekly feedback, so that you are well prepared for assessments and end of placement reports;
- help you to address your own learning agenda as well as that required by the course.

Pause now to think about how you can establish an early rapport with your mentor. Make a list of things that you could do and give a short rationale for each.

We share some of our ideas at the end of the chapter.

The working relationship with the mentor should be one of trust, purposeful work and mutual respect. Mentors expect students to arrive ready and eager to learn in the placement setting. The relationship has to grow, though, and not all mentorship relationships are equally satisfying. It is possible that you will complete some placements where you feel that you did not achieve a good rapport with your mentor. The placement may still have been a success – you passed the assessments and gained new insights, but it was much harder work than one where the mentor seemed enthusiastic, receptive to your enquiries and ready to gently challenge your assumptions. Search for, savour and celebrate the exceptional working relationships with mentors and acknowledge your own hard work with the less satisfying ones. Then ask some reflective questions. Could you have approached matters differently? Sometimes circumstances are against you both, for instance where staff sickness disrupts the continuity of your supervision.

As the working relationship develops, opportunities exist to deepen understanding between you and to begin to explore what it means to work as a nurse. Table 6.2 describes some of those opportunities and includes reflections from Gina on what does or doesn't seem to help.

Table 6.2: Mentorship-linked learning opportunities.

Learning opportunity	Gina's notes
Evaluating your own performance, for example associated with a clinical procedure.	*It is a mentor's duty to give you honest feedback on your performance, but sometimes you get the best of this when you ask for their comments. You need to indicate that you're ready to hear constructive criticism.*
Sharing some doubts about your ability or understanding.	*You pay the mentor a compliment when you confide a doubt, and the best of them really appreciate this. I did so concerning my maths and the calculation of drugs. My reward was a series of mini teach-ins that boosted my confidence.*
Talking honestly about a team relationship that worries you.	*You won't get on with every member of the team. I think that it's good to try to resolve issues in the placement if possible. In one instance, the mentor was able to explain why a consultant seemed brusque and I felt reassured that I wasn't doing something wrong. Remember, though, you cannot expect the mentor to help you if the discussion remains completely secret. The mentor might need to represent your concerns elsewhere.*
Expressing some hopes and aspirations about future nursing work.	*I hadn't thought about this, but you're right! We need to keep dreaming. It helps us keep going when times seem tough. There were mentors who encouraged career aspirations.*
Securing recommended reading.	*Yes. I have even been loaned books and articles by a considerate mentor. But, remember, the library doesn't shut because you have gone on a placement.*
Celebrating your first successes.	*The first person to congratulate me after I passed my placement report was my mentor. It wasn't a perfect performance, but the mentor said to me, 'Do you realise how rare it is to achieve such warm comments from so many different professionals?'*
Appraising what needs to be done to meet objectives, to pass assessment.	*Definitely. The end report should never be a surprise and, if you're open with your mentor, you will get lots of warning about what needs improvement.*

Managing assessment

We come, then, to assessment. Reports are linked to clinical placements and these cover matters such as the development of your skills, the attitudes that you demonstrate in practice, your commitment to nursing care and the gains made in your knowledge there (Stuart, 2007). In previous times assessment was formalised as a series of events, and these were linked to key tasks such as the medicine round. Today, assessment is said to be 'continuous' and we need to consider the psychology of this. The first thought that many students have is just how daunting it seems: 'During a clinical placement I am likely to make many mistakes, say a number of "wrong things" and inevitably alienate someone!' Continuous assessment highlights how vulnerable it can seem to be a student.

However, there has to be judgement on performance, and this remains an issue for qualified nurses as well. Annual staff appraisals, complaints by patients and reviews by auditors are all part of professional life. Assessments that are made of your performance are mediated by an understanding of your stage of training and the learning objectives set; they comprise inputs from a number of staff members and take account of both the 'good days' and the 'bad days' of your time in placement. The staff are interested in your learning, and your response to guidance. While you might demonstrate shortfalls in skill or knowledge, these can often be compensated for by a willingness to receive instruction. What will make it very difficult for mentors and others to pass a student on their placement are shortfalls in skill and/or knowledge, combined with a refusal on the part of a student to change.

To help you manage assessment, then, you need to be critical of your own performance and to search for gaps in your skill or knowledge. You will need to recognise misconceptions that are not serving you well. Such a personal audit of week-by-week performance will then enable you to seek the guidance of your mentor and, at the earliest possible point, to start correcting any shortfalls and building on your successes. The following represent a series of week-by-week questions that might help you to evaluate your progress.

- What do you think was the best of my work this week and what still needed improvement? (Notice the search for both. It helps to receive praise as well as constructive criticism. Recognition of effort and attentiveness will stand you in good stead.)
- If you were to suggest one focus for improving my practice next week, what would that be and why? (Sometimes it is important to focus on a specific area and, if you can demonstrate a major improvement here, you will show your ability to reflect and develop.)
- How do you think it feels for a patient to be nursed by me? (This is a bold question, but patient experience is everything. An exploration of what represents quality there can be very useful.)
- I've written down three things that I think I'm good at and three things where I think I could do better. Would you check whether I have made good choices? (Here you are using the 'check my speculation' approach. It is a powerful approach because it shows your openness to change and reveals where you think there could be problems. At worst, the mentor will gently point out your misconceptions and you can refocus your efforts. At best, you are told honestly that you underestimate yourself in several regards.)

Activity 6.5 *Reflection*

Have you, in association with a clinical placement, ever asked any of the above questions or something similar? What was the response that you received and did it help you to take charge of the learning that you did next? If you haven't asked such questions, or feel that it would be difficult to do so, what are the possible costs of not understanding how others see your learning work in the clinical area?

We share brief points on this at the end of the chapter.

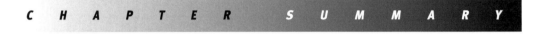

C H A P T E R   S U M M A R Y

Looking back over this chapter, we hope that you go away from it with several key messages. The first is that learning in clinical practice is different and that you must be an active and organised learner. You help shape the learning experience by working with your mentor and using steps such as those described in Figure 6.1. Learning in clinical practice need not seem chaotic, confusing and inaccessible, if you think critically about what you encounter and continue to ask questions about what you experience and achieve. In clinical practice you cannot easily separate out the emotions that attend new experiences, and it is part of your learning work to accommodate these. Pausing to mull these over, alongside your first interpretation of events, will enable you to ask sensible questions later on. It takes time to resolve emotional differences between what you think should be and what could be – between *my way* and *their way*.

A cycle of inquisitive questions, however, will not by and of themselves guarantee learning. You will need to invite questions and challenges from others. You need to search out and then carefully consider the feedback that you receive. It can seem bruising to face a criticism about something that you thought you were already good at, but remember, contexts change and what worked in one place might not be appropriate in another. Nursing is a craft, an art and a profession that works within contexts. Mentors in particular do not give critical feedback lightly, mindful as they are of how vulnerable learners can feel. The feedback will usually be carefully considered and supported afterwards with a review of what might improve matters.

Forming a good working relationship with your mentor significantly increases your learning opportunities. In a trusting relationship there is scope to express doubts and to confront long-held fears. You may, like Gina, resolve a difficulty that liberates your learning throughout the rest of the course. Building a rapport with your mentor offers the prospect of a placement that not only teaches you a great deal, but that provides you with a great deal of learning pleasure.

Activities: brief outline answers and reflections

Activity 6.1: Reflection (page 77)

It is hard for students to switch from campus enquiry to clinical enquiry, because the two areas have different traditions of learning. In the first, the student is encouraged to be challenging, inquisitive and discursive, and sometimes to test ideas and ideals in open debate. Learning seems less deferential, as befits the campus setting and the historical role of universities, where the boundaries of knowledge are tested. The clinical learning environment is different, though, and is, in many regards, more formal and understandably referenced against risk management, professional integrity and the reputation of clinical teams. In moving between the two, you will need to change your frame of reference, respecting the different traditions. It is not that one is better than the other, but rather that each context affects the manner of enquiry. Understand the norms in each and learning becomes more productive.

Activity 6.3: Critical thinking (page 81)

We argue that there are several situations where a clear appreciation of the process of learning – what you are trying to do and how this is being achieved – materially improves your chances of success and your enjoyment of study. One of those is research projects, where the researcher has to make sense of data and ask the right questions to secure defensible conclusions. The first and most profound, though, is learning in clinical practice. If you don't think in clear, strategic terms, you are likely to feel bewildered by experiences, few of which seem to add up coherently to an explanation of what nurses do. What seemed to work in one situation didn't in another. What was acceptable in one context, seemed reprehensible in another. What was taught in the lecture theatre seems misplaced when we consider nursing practice. We can only engage with such discrepancies and gain confidence if we develop an approach to learning that is clearly about sense-making. We accept uncertainty, allow information to accumulate and ask relevant questions to test out our speculations. We understand the compromises reached, discover what our position on a subject is and learn to live with the complexity and sometimes the idiosyncrasies of practice.

Activity 6.4: Communication (page 81)

Here are four ideas.

- Attend carefully to the opening briefing shared by your mentor, making notes as appropriate.
- Ask the mentor about what other students have enjoyed or found difficult as regards the clinical placement. In doing so, you enable the mentor to talk about their experience, which is something that you wish to tap into.
- Keep all your appointments. Mentors are busy people and have heavy clinical responsibilities, so you should make good use of what they offer.
- Check with your mentor at the outset the best times to ask questions. If you are able to discuss Figure 6.1, your mentor should feel reassured that you are an enthusiastic, inquisitive but considerate student.

Activity 6.5: Reflection (page 84)

Failing to seek feedback has several possible consequences. You may continue blindly with practice that, while not dangerous, remains less than considerate. You may develop a reputation for arrogance and face a future shock when you are confronted about your attitude. Failing to examine your shortfalls may mean that you limit future learning. Because you don't realise that you are missing an insight, you use your assumptions as a basis for future thinking and the difficulty becomes compounded. You may, of course, fail the clinical placement.

Knowledge review

1. Below, we draw some analogies regarding the process of learning in clinical placements. Which is the one that you should adopt given your reading of the above chapter?
   a. Learning here is like mining – you go in and extract what is needed.
   b. Learning here is a bit like begging – you need to hold up your bowl for what comes your way.
   c. Learning here is like a journey – you try to observe things along the way, communicating with those who know the path.
   d. Learning here is a contest – others don't want you to know and you have to overcome that.

Now answer the following three questions.

2. Why is it important to work at building a good rapport with your mentor?
3. What happens between observing practice and reformulating what you will do in the future?
4. Why is continuous assessment in clinical practice less daunting than you might first imagine?

Further reading

Dougherty, L and Lister, S (2008) *The Royal Marsden Hospital Manual of Clinical Nursing Procedures,* 7th edition. Chichester: Wiley Blackwell.
Your work in clinical placements will quickly alert you to variances in clinical procedures and will prompt questions about why they are carried out in particular ways. This well-established textbook lays bare the thinking behind those adopted at a famous London hospital. We recommend that you read this book as an example of what can benchmark clinical procedures, and then consider what it teaches you about investigating the rationale for how and why things are done in a particular way.

Endacott, R, Jevon, P and Cooper, S (2009) *Clinical Nursing Skills, Core and Advanced.* Oxford: Oxford University Press.
Much of what you learn in clinical practice is associated with clinical skills. This textbook offers an up-to-date review of skills, each of which is underpinned by the ability to think and reflect in a coherent way. Studying the differences between core and advanced skills provides excellent insights into the ways in which critical thinking operates at these different levels.

Sharples, K (2009) *Learning to Learn in Nursing Practice.* Exeter: Learning Matters.
Our sister volume provides further in-depth discussion of the process of learning within the clinical setting, and reminds the reader about the ethical, educational and historical context of such learning. There is further material here on working with a mentor and preparing for your placement.

Useful websites

http://ezinearticles.com/?Nine-Reasons-Why-Mentoring-Matters-to-You&id=68604
Kevin Eikenberry (undated) Nine reasons why mentoring matters to you, EzineArticles.com
This site offers a simple aide-memoire on the benefits of being a mentor – something that might help sustain the hard-pressed practitioner who serves in this role.

www.mentoringdimensions.com
Mentoring Dimensions (Ann Darwin), MARC Management and Research Centre
The personalities or dispositions of mentors can be important in whether they form good working relationships with others. This business-based site provides a chance for mentors to self-calculate their strengths and weaknesses on different mentoring dimensions (free to use).

Chapter 7

Making use of electronic media

NMC Standards for Pre-registration Nursing Education (2010)

Because the subject matter covered by electronic media varies widely, there are no specific standards to link to. The skills covered in this chapter underpin how you successfully learn and achieve all the standards, within the environment of electronic media.

Chapter aims

By the end of this chapter you will be able to:

*   summarise the ways in which electronic media communication influences critical thinking;
*   identify the ways in which electronic media might enhance the quality of your learning;
*   explore personal feelings, aspirations and concerns regarding the use of electronic media within your course of studies;
*   identify ways in which tutors provide feedback on assignments and how this could be used;
*   prepare appropriate contributions to electronic forums associated with your course of studies.

Introduction

We have seen in preceding chapters how the environment in which we learn plays a role in shaping our thinking. In the clinical setting, for instance, the way in which we ask questions is influenced by the nature of the clinical work. In workshops, thinking is moulded by the exercises that we engage in. Learning to use the current electronic media is as much a part of successful learning as is command of a subject or practice skill. We need to realise what opportunities the media offer.

Electronic media are widely used within nursing courses to support student learning, networking and skills development. If you complete your studies at a distance, the part played by electronic media may be even greater. Email, electronic conference forums, wikis and electronic noticeboards and cafés have become a significant part of the course experience. You may, for example, get feedback on assignments by email, and perhaps engage in debates online.

In this chapter, we examine what is involved in learning using different electronic media and make suggestions about how you can derive benefit from them. We will acknowledge some of the anxieties associated with the use of these media and explore the ways in which they advance your ability to think critically. To illustrate critical thinking and reflection in action we will refer to two case studies. The first of these is the handling of emailed assignment feedback. The second relates to electronic forums and concerns the development of arguments around best nursing practice.

Messages and the media

Just how important learning media are to nurse education can be illustrated with some items from an imaginary time capsule. Imagine that you have dug the capsule up and, within it, you find:

- a 1960s' medical-surgical nursing textbook;
- a chalkboard and a set of chalks;
- an overhead projector and some acetates;
- a computer-based instruction program that teaches you the nursing process;
- a file containing discussions from an online course forum.

Activity 7.1   *Reflection*

Look at the above items and decide how you think each of these may have shaped the teaching and learning of nursing. More profoundly still, do you think that they also influence how we as nurses think and reflect?

As this activity is based on your own reflection, there is no answer at the end of the chapter.

During the 1960s, medical-surgical nursing textbooks were a key resource in the training of nurses. Typically, the chapters were divided into accounts of illnesses, their treatment and then the associated nursing care. There was a lot of emphasis on nursing procedures and tasks, and it was accepted that nursing care was largely dictated by the treatment ordered by a doctor. Were you to read such a textbook today, you might remark how formulaic the care seemed. Nurses were instructed to think, but did so within carefully prescribed boundaries.

You may have already encountered teaching using a chalkboard or perhaps a whiteboard. What is significant about it, though, is the way it concentrates learning on the teacher. 'Chalk and talk' teaching involved the teacher lecturing an audience and periodically placing figures or lists of points on the board that the student was required to copy down. While students could be invited to use the chalk- or whiteboard them-selves, teaching was usually in one direction – from teacher to student.

Overhead projectors caused similar problems. Lessons were determined by what was prepared on the acetates that were placed on the machine projecting images on to a screen. The tutor could swop and/or reorder the sequence of acetates, but the agenda for what was to be taught was largely pre-set. Scope remained open (as before) for conversation, but the breadth and depth of critical thinking and reflection were usually still constrained by the mindset of delivering the required content of the session. This same thinking, based on delivery of required information, was still influential in the early computer-based instruction programs. As a student you would work through the series of on-screen pages, complete the simple tests that appeared periodically, and then finish the lesson, perhaps noting at the end your final score.

It is the file of the online forum discussions, however, that represents a significant departure in terms of learning and teaching. Depending on how the forum is run, there is scope here for students as well as tutors to set agendas, for students to lead sections of discussion, and for the whole to be based solidly upon discourse. While tutors may well have 'posted' (positioned) resources here (such as hyperlink connections to important library materials), and moderate the conversation in terms of acceptable contributions, the learning is strongly centred on shared reasoning. If all the other items within the time capsule nurtured private learning, the online forum expected communal and arguably expansive learning (that is, learning that demonstrates the evolution of ideas, arguments and reflections, shared by other members of the group, and that remain on record in a way that other forms of teaching often do not). It was necessary to think aloud.

Activity 7.2   *Reflection*

Having completed Activity 7.1, reflect now on your feelings about the different learning styles that seem to be demanded in association with the media discussed above. Do you think of yourself as someone who is more comfortable learning privately or publically? Being honest about these reflections is important, because it influences what you take from electronic learning media within your course.

We share some reflections of our own at the end of the chapter.

Email

Your use of electronic media (e.g., Facebook, Twitter, mail-order sites) in the past may have been linked to things such as social networking, online shopping and text messaging using a mobile phone. Students vary widely in their electronic media experience and older students may feel less electronic media 'savvy' than their younger peers. Upon joining your course, though, it is likely that you will be linked to a course webpage within the university and have an email account set up for you so that you can communicate more flexibly with your tutor, the library and study group colleagues. Email extends the campus in significant ways, even before we begin to outline the more sophisticated media. Through email you may receive a 'study group message' from your tutor that is broadcast to the group as a whole. Using email you might be encouraged to develop a 'study buddy' working relationship with one or more other students. Sometimes a more senior student is asked to mentor a more junior learner and email aids communication.

Just as there is etiquette associated with the use of electronic forums ('netiquette'), so there is one associated with the use of email for educational purposes. Beyond the usual caution that to type in CAPITALS is rude (it equates to shouting), there are other, equally important, rules associated with what is and isn't to be discussed using an email. For example, you may discuss a draft piece of coursework with your tutor or personal tutor by email, but to do so with a study buddy might be to risk censure. This is because of the university rules concerning academic collusion and the need to ensure that work is not plagiarised. It is wise, then, to check university rules associated with academic collaboration and to consider what this means for your use of emails while at university.

Wikis

You may not have encountered a wiki before joining your course, but it can simply be described as an electronic space where individuals make contributions that add to the understanding of a subject (Leuf and Cunningham, 2002). Individuals type their entry to the wiki in a text box, check what they have written and then post it to the wiki space on the course webpage. The purpose of a wiki is to add layers of information – extra interpretations of what has been posted as the subject of the wiki. So, for example, your tutor may have invited the study group to contribute examples and definitions of the term 'rehabilitation'. In this way, as each of you adds a small contribution (typically a paragraph or so), an extended definition of the concept emerges, which might later be discussed as part of a tutorial. The wiki remains online as a reference resource for you and others to draw on later.

Activity 7.3   *Critical thinking*

Make a few notes on the following.

- What are the attractions and responsibilities associated with wikis?
- Are they useful as a means of helping you to develop your own reasoning?

We have shared some of our own reflections at the end of the chapter.

Electronic forums

Most courses offer electronic forums, which are places where students and tutors can communicate with one another, either asynchronously (i.e., over time) or synchronously (i.e., at a designated time when all participants are asked to be online together, so that communication is more immediate). As with wikis, you access the relevant electronic forum using your student identification number and individual password, a process that ensures the relative privacy of discussions within that space. At the informal end of the spectrum, electronic forums are designated 'cafés' and you are free to discuss a wide range of topics connected to university life. At the more formal end of the spectrum, individual forum discussions are connected to course modules and postings made there may demonstrate your 'attendance' or even contribute to course marks achieved.

In the formal forums, a series of individual discussions is initiated (often by the tutor) and, as each student adds responses of their own, a 'thread' develops. At different points the tutor may tidy up the thread, editing material so as to ensure that the final record of discussion remains comprehensible to students. Also, in editing the thread, work is undertaken to ensure accessibility. It is not done to change your thoughts or points, save only where you post something that goes beyond what is allowed by the university as being respectful to others.

- Given the above description of electronic forums and the posting of messages there, how does this differ from the conversations that you share face to face?
- What are the advantages and the disadvantages of this, and how might it affect the way that you represent your thinking to others?

We will be sharing a student response to this activity on page 94.

Making good use of feedback

We come now to the first of two case studies within this chapter and one designed to help you to make the best use of electronic media to develop your learning. As part of your coursework it is possible that you will submit both formative assignments (those that aren't awarded a grade) and summative assignments (those that do secure a grade) electronically to your tutor and receive your feedback in a similarly paper-free way. Electronic submission has the advantage that you can obtain a track record of the assignment being submitted on time. Also, you have more time to complete the work (you don't hard copy mail assignments or wait until a study day to hand them in). One of the other key advantages of an electronically submitted assignment is that the tutor can give you both summary feedback (as an end-of-work commentary) and feedback in the form of textual annotations that you can read as part of an attachment emailed back to you (see Figure 7.1). This figure illustrates two forms of feedback on a single paragraph extract from a student's assignment answer.

In Figure 7.1 there are two forms of feedback on offer. The first is called 'track change' and is presented here as underlined text that appears within the body of the

Figure 7.1: Examples of track change and margin note commentary feedback.

Children have particular difficulties expressing pain. Younger ones have a more limited vocabulary to describe the pain and may use general terms like 'tummy' to refer to its location. They don't have a clear sense of time and may struggle to describe the duration of the pain. MacGrath (1989)[McGrath (1990) in your reference list[ER1]] explains that nurses have to use parents to help interpret the pain. Parents are familiar with the way in which a child expresses themselves and can help determine whether pain may be a problem, for example when the child seems distracted and unable to concentrate on what they are doing[ER2]. Children have just as much pain as the rest of us and it's wrong to assume that they don't feel pain in the same way as adults[You need a reference here and perhaps to consider making this a separate paragraph. This paragraph is all about the expression of pain and your last point is about the incidence or nature of pain encountered].

Comment [ER1]: Are there more recent references that you could use?

Comment [ER2]: Do you think there are any circumstances when we need to be more cautious about relying upon a parent to help interpret a child's pain? If you are unsure, why not look up 'Munchausen by proxy' syndrome?

essay work. In the first instance, track change has been used to correct the presentation of a reference. The adjustment shows the correct spelling of the author name and queries the date of publication. In the second track change, the tutor provides guidance on both the referencing of the work and the planning of coherent paragraphs. Each paragraph should have a distinctive subject. The second form of feedback consists of margin annotations. ER in this instance stands for 'educational reviewer', although initials can be changed to reflect the name of the tutor. ER doesn't stand for 'error', because some margin annotations can be used to congratulate you on your work: 'Michelle, this is excellent, you summarise the theory with great skill!'

While the volume and complexity of written feedback on an assignment answer may vary, good feedback remains unambiguous. There are no unexplained ?s and !s dotted around that leave you to guess what the tutor means. The question then remains: what purpose is the feedback fulfilling, and how will you make sense of it and what will you do next?

The purpose of feedback

One purpose of feedback is to correct a misapprehension, whether that concerns a reference, a drug calculation or an assertion about ethical care. Corrections are often handled using track changes, with the tutor either deleting something and inserting the correct material, or commenting on the deficits. But other feedback may have a more subtle function. Comment ER1 in Figure 7.1 is designed to prompt some further thought and enquiry. While this form of challenge is designed to help you to improve work, other challenges are more rhetorical and are designed to illustrate the way in which the tutor is 'thinking aloud' beside you (ER2). Tutors don't invariably expect you to respond to such remarks, but leave them for further consideration. On occasions, the margin commentary is intentionally provocative as well as rhetorical, as in this example: 'Perhaps we are naive to imagine that any of us can completely assess the pain of another. Pain is bound up with private experiences, memories and fears. I wonder what you think?'

In these ways, the feedback that you receive within a returned assignment becomes a delayed conversation. The tutor indicates, 'This is what I noticed, this is where I wish to guide you and here is where reflections could go a little further.' At best, feedback starts to model critical thinking for you, and reviews the state of current knowledge as well as your answer to a set question.

Making sense of feedback

We need, then, to make sense of the tutor's feedback. Does it require a response on my part? Does it prompt some new work for me? Am I invited to request some additional help? However important a coursework mark or grade might seem (and we note this first of all, don't we?), the commentary that accompanies your assignment answer is the most useful of all. Even if you have achieved a good mark, there is always something more to glean from the commentary provided. Why is this a good essay? Seeing the pass mark, noting the warm tone of the tutor's feedback and heaving a sigh of relief are not enough. You need to ascertain what the tutor thinks you have learned here and what could remain to be achieved.

Doing something with feedback

While, logistically, tutors supporting large student groups cannot enter into protracted dialogue with every student, there is a strong case for corresponding further with your tutor in the following circumstances.

- Where you have secured a poor grade and where the commentary suggests that you have misunderstood the question.
- Where the commentary suggests a significant gap in your subject knowledge (that gap may prove important in later assessments).
- Where the feedback has posed new questions to you (you wish to ask the tutor to help clarify a matter).
- Where the tutor has suggested other possible lines of enquiry.

It is understandable to worry that you may inconvenience a busy tutor, but if they signal the above things, they really do welcome contact with you. At this point you need conviction about the purpose of the assignment. Yes, it may be a test of your progress and come with a grade, but it is also part of learning too. The conversations that follow on from the assignment feedback will help you to develop your powers of discrimination and argument formation.

Activity 7.5   *Reflection*

Reflect now on any assignment feedback that you have received to date and answer the following question.

- Did I use this to help develop my critical thinking/reflective practice?

If the answer is no, decide next why that was.

- Did the electronic form of communication put you off – making it seem impersonal?
- Or, on the contrary, did it make receiving feedback easier?
- What have you perhaps lost by not seizing this opportunity?

As this activity is based on your own reflection, there is no answer at the end of the chapter.

Making arguments in the forum

Our second example of electronic media-mediated learning concerns the use of electronic forums. Tutors use these forums for various purposes, including the development of study group conversations (learning from one another), as a means of collecting together a range of views, and as a means of helping you to track changes in your collective thinking (tutors can archive forum discussions and later invite your group to examine changes in reasoning). Making contributions to the forum, and especially arguments online, can seem more difficult, though. We asked Fatima to complete Activity 7.4 (see page 92) and here are some of her reflections on contributing to forums:

> I have enjoyed the different forums that we shared during the course so far. To read other people's ideas and to have them there, at midnight if you wished, is something that I never thought would be possible. But posting my ideas was more difficult. It was easy to support someone else, to say 'yes I agree', but more difficult to make a case, to suggest something of my own. I found myself thinking, 'this is not polite, to insist in this way to my colleagues.' My personal tutor smiled

and noted that in my clinical placement I was described as 'a bit quiet'. She was right, I have not been brought up to assert myself and I know that nurses must do that. But there is a difference between class and computer. In class I can say things. I make my views heard. In the computer, though, the words last forever; they are there on screen and, just as I can read other people's words, so they can read mine. I feel exposed by that and worry that, if my words seem unwise, I will suffer.

Fatima's reflections are familiar to tutors. As another student once put it, 'Debating in the forum is like making a maiden speech in Parliament. An audience is listening to you and it will be recorded.' However, making arguments is necessary if you are to advance your thinking. There is a need to formulate arguments and to test them with supportive peers and an empathetic tutor. Happily, the system for posting forum messages involves composition and there is a chance to review your posting before it is electronically submitted. While most students do this to check their grammar and syntax (worrying about presentation), the greatest benefit of the pre-submission check is being able to consider whether your points seem coherent and clear. No one in the forum expects perfection, especially in a synchronous discussion, where postings happen a little faster. No one anticipates that their comments will always be supported either. Just as in other conversations, there will be some good points made and some that seem more questionable. Making a clear argument, though, is something that we can practise when we edit messages before they are posted.

Activity 7.6   *Critical thinking*

Imagine now that you are engaged in a forum discussion about the right (or otherwise) of individuals to end their own lives. The last posting made by another student expresses a deeply held religious conviction that patients should not exercise such a right and that, to do so, relieves healthcare practitioners of the responsibility to search for and deliver quality of life support measures. Now it is your turn to offer something. Consider the three short arguments below and decide which, if any, you might post to the forum. We discuss the merits of each below, but encourage you to evaluate them first as this will help you consider how to prepare postings to forums. Whether you support one or any of these postings will depend in part on whether you are clear on your views concerning end-of-life decisions.

1. I can see Susan's point regarding who should have the right to curtail a life, but it is fair to observe that significant numbers of people do not express a religious conviction and question whether there is an absolute law here. We might need to remember other healthcare philosophy that we operate with. Perhaps there is a link to consumerism. If we require patients to make choices in other areas, for instance as regards medication, why are they not capable of making such decisions about death?

2. One of the things that we wrestle with is how patients' decisions make us feel. Their actions seem to reflect on us. 'I ended my life because you couldn't help me.' This seems a terrible thing and yet these are views we can imagine patients holding. In another year they might have other choices available to them.

3. The media debate concerning this topic is often about the intentions of those who facilitate death. If there are inheritance benefits being sought, or if the death of the person simply makes life more convenient for others, ending a life undermines all that is dignified in society. If the decision is truthfully about the relief of suffering, and acknowledges that quality of life has gone, perhaps we have to support carers.

As this discussion continues in the text, there is no answer at the end of the chapter.

We start by stating that this is a very powerful debate and one that would only be undertaken by confident students. It is not a place where a new student would be expected to start! The formulation of an argument here, however, is shaped by:

- concerns about what you think and wish to convey (being genuine about your own beliefs);
- issues concerning how this will seem to others (audience reaction);
- clarity of what you wish to convey (easy or difficult);
- whether you wish to make a new point or contest a previous one;
- coherence (can I demonstrate a reasoned point?).

Response (1) above gently contests the point made by Susan, noting that it is the beliefs of the individual patient, as much as those of the practitioner, that should help determine how end-of-life decisions are made. The point is well reasoned. If patients have responsibilities as healthcare consumers, they also have rights. The argument could be developed further, but it is clear. If we were making this argument, though, we might end with an invitation that shows that we are posting in speculative mode: 'Does anyone else hold views on this? I'm just searching through this idea about how being a consumer affects things here.' What is important is that the argument made needs to be measured and open to speculation by others, otherwise the point made could seem bigoted. The person posting this argument feels comfortable that they are expressing an authentic position (one that highlights individuality), and that their point is coherent (if patients have responsibilities as consumers, they should have rights too).

Response (2) seems tangential to the point made regarding religious convictions and end-of-life decisions. It acknowledges our discomforts about such decisions and illuminates the problem, without necessarily expressing the student's position. It might express an 'I simply don't know' perspective. Your position doesn't instantly have to be shared in the first posting – it could be something that you edge towards through discussion. There is nothing wrong with such contributions to a forum, as they offer extra dimensions to think about. Later, the tutor may sum up these considerations and pose some new questions.

Response (3) seems to move on to a new area of argument – that of consequences and carers. What if relatives or friends help someone to die? The link to the current point about rights is there, but is not as direct as we might expect. Had you made this argument, it would certainly still be welcomed as thoughtful and reflective. Later, though, it might be moved to another discussion – one associated with how we should see the role of the lay carer. What is important here is that new points should be targeted towards the discussion topic. It is harder for others to make use of your argument if it wanders elsewhere.

What can we say, then, about the business of making arguments within electronic forums? First, it seems necessary to accept that forums are not the same sorts of conversations that we share elsewhere. While they are collegiate, they aren't transient. They leave a record and it is for this reason that you will naturally wish to compose your arguments carefully. Second, successful forums are permissive and allow that ideas and arguments will develop within and through them. You will make several postings and the clarity of matters will improve as the group takes stock of what has been posted. It is OK to 'feel your way' in these matters. Your tutor has a key role here, helping to sum up points. Third, discussions held there are not and should not be reputation busters. Your tutor should make this clear at the outset, otherwise trust will not grow within the study group. Provided basic etiquette guidelines are followed, the forum remains a place for speculation and the practising of arguments.

You are likely to enrich your critical thinking by recognising the multiple perspectives that exist on a subject within the forum. Your views will not necessarily be those of others and the tutor does not relieve you of this uncertainty by stating that 'nursing has this view'. You will develop your reasoning ability because you have to formulate points that others can understand and relate to. Notice, for example, the connection made to consumerism in response (1) above. This student reminds companions that, if we subscribe to a consumerist philosophy, we cannot so easily abandon the free choice principle in the matter of end-of-life decisions. It may take practice to represent such points, drawing on your observations and experience, but the effort that you put in here may well pay dividends later in writing assignment answers.

CHAPTER SUMMARY

In this chapter we began with the argument that communication media have an important influence on the messages shared, and we hope that we have proven this point. The way you reason using electronic media will be different from reasoning in class. This is not to suggest, however, that the media in some way undermine the critical thinking and reflection that can operate here. The quality of feedback possible with an electronically submitted assignment, and the depth of debate possible within an electronic forum, both offer rich opportunities. The very fact that you can access conversations at times to suit you, and that there is space to compose your answers with care that is not available in a real-time face-to-face conversation, highlights the opportunities to develop critical thinking here. Electronic media make a major contribution to 'thinking time'; they prompt you to reflect before you speak and this is valuable.

Electronic media, however, are not without their challenges and you may have observed through the activities within this chapter just how strange this communication can seem. For some, it feels artificial, especially if students are more private and contemplative in nature. Tutors are becoming adept, though, in creating welcoming and supportive electronic learning environments. They recognise the anxieties that can lurk as you prepare your first postings, and they know that to contribute to something that remains 'on record' undermines the confidence of some. Acknowledging these concerns, they arrange feedback and summarise discussions in ways that demonstrate tolerance, an appreciation of your efforts and a commitment to imaginative new ways to learn.

Activities: brief outline answers and reflections

Activity 7.2: Reflection (page 90)

Our anecdotal experience is that students tend towards a preference for either private learning or a more communal, public form of learning. If you prefer a more private form of learning, some of the work associated with electronic media might seem onerous. This is not to suggest that one learning style is correct, normal or mandatory. Each has its strengths. Within nursing, though, and especially, as we have seen in Chapter 6, within clinical learning environments, communal learning is rewarded and valued. Nurses need to 'reason aloud' as part of working towards shared solutions. For this reason, more communal forms of learning have an important part to play.

Activity 7.3: Critical thinking (page 91)

Attractions of the wiki

- The study group can develop its own resource of communal information.
- Wikis can be used to develop a glossary of key terms associated with your course.
- Because many people contribute to wikis, no single person dominates the learning.
- Wikis remain readily available; you can return to them again and again (e.g., when revising for examinations).

Responsibilities of the wiki

- Wikis only work if enough students make entries.
- What you contribute should be factually accurate.
- Wikis are not a debating chamber – others may contribute things that you disagree with. Providing that the information contained there is factually correct, you will need to show tolerance.

Knowledge review

To help you check your command of this chapter, answer the following questions.

1. What evidence might you point to in support of the claim that the media of learning affect your critical thinking?
2. What do you think are the key benefits of receiving feedback on your coursework assignments in an electronic form?
3. What is there to be gained from making contributions in an electronic forum?
4. What are the considerations to take into account when composing contributions to an electronic course forum?

Further reading

Littlejohn, A and Pegler, C (2007) *Preparing for Blended e-Learning*. Abingdon: Routledge.

This is predominantly a book for the blended learning course designer and tutor, although the discussions are accessible enough for the student interested in learning as a process within this medium. The work majors on the design of more interactive forms of learning within the medium and the challenges that designers can face here.

Mason, R and Rennie, F (2006) *E-Learning: The key concepts*. Abingdon: Routledge.
This is a very short guide to e-learning, and particularly to the terminology that you may encounter there. It is especially useful for students who discover that they enjoy this medium and wish to explore the approach further.

Santy, J and Smith, L (2007) *Being an e-Learner in Health and Social Care: A student's guide*. Abingdon: Routledge.
This is a comprehensive guide to a range of issues associated with e-learning within healthcare and includes an important chapter about professional issues and discussions online. The book clarifies the role of the tutor and the expectations made of students, highlighting what has so far been developed in this approach to learning.

Useful website

www.bbc.co.uk/learning (BBC Learning)
It can seem daunting to learn online in a subject where your professional reputation is at stake. For that reason we thoroughly recommend that you indulge yourself at the BBC, sampling video clips and other online learning resources that come from the archives there. This shows you what fun an online learning environment can be and helps build confidence as you return to nursing studies.

Expressing critical thought and reflection

Chapter 8

Writing the analytical essay

NMC Standards for Pre-registration Nursing Education (2010)

Because the subject matter covered in analytical essays varies widely, there are no specific standards to link to. The skills covered in this chapter underpin how you successfully learn and achieve all the standards, within the context of analytical essay writing.

Chapter aims

By the end of this chapter you will be able to:

- determine clearly the purpose of the analytical essays you are asked to write;
- identify the cases presented by others or the one that you will deliberate on;
- adopt a clear position on the case within your analytical essay;
- select relevant evidence and link this to arguments within your written work;
- demonstrate more speculative and scholarly ways of writing in your essays;
- prepare conclusions that both sum up previous text and demonstrate what you deduce from it.

Introduction

During the course of your studies you will write a series of analytical essays, some of which you will tackle under examination conditions. No one assumes that what you achieve in examinations will necessarily be as good as what is managed within coursework. Without prior notification of the topics to be covered, you will write to best possible effect using your memory and any permitted notes. Time constraints limit your ability to plan, so you will need to use the precepts of critical thinking that you were introduced to in Chapter 1, and remember the basic structure of an answer, as explored in Chapter 3.

In this chapter, we combine our previous teaching on critical thinking and writing, and apply this to analytical essays. We consider the purposes to which the analytical essay is put and highlight the importance of establishing clarity of thought, and your position, before you start writing. We review how best to discriminate what should be included in the essay, and then the use of arguments that demonstrate your ability to weigh the merits and limitations of a case. We revisit how best to sum up the essay within the conclusion and make the point that success here consists of much more than simply repeating what has been presented earlier in the paper.

To help you to examine these points in some depth, we have arranged for an example analytical essay (kindly supplied by Stewart, one of the four students associated with this book) to be made available on the Learning Matters website (**www.learningmatters.co.uk/nursing**). You can learn much from this chapter without referring to that resource, but we think it offers valuable examples of critical writing in action. Stewart's essay is not perfect, neither is it intended to become a template for exactly how you should write. The work focuses on one subject – a review of how nurses make use of different sorts of evidence. But it enables us to discuss analytical writing in the context of a specific question. At the point that this essay was written, Stewart was nearing the end of his course. You should not assume that this is a standard to be achieved from the outset of study. Read it, therefore, with a view to identifying what it can teach you about technique, and not as a comparison with your own work!

The purpose of analytical essays

Analytical essays are set for different purposes. The first of these is to test your understanding of a given subject and your ability to make a series of well-informed judgements about it (the evaluative essay). Such essays are frequently set as a review of the literature, research reports or healthcare policies. Examiners wish to understand whether you have a clear grasp of what others have argued, and whether you have developed a clear perspective of your own. The second purpose of the analytical essay is to move forward from this, to assess your strategic thinking: what would you do next and why? These sorts of essays are frequently presented in the form of patient case studies, and here you would combine the declarative, procedural, knowledge and decision-making components of critical thinking discussed in Chapter 1 (the strategic essay). The third purpose of analytical essays is to test your ability to confront conundrums or to examine professional ethos (the philosophical essay). Sometimes there is no obviously right or straightforward answer, and no neat solution, and the nurse has to manage a situation as it is. Papers about ethical dilemmas may be of this kind. A command of care philosophy and ethics is important if you are to cope with the stresses of healthcare practice. Examiners want to know that you grasp the complexity of issues and the processes that will help you deal with these.

Activity 8.1   *Critical thinking*

Below are some essay assignment questions or instructions. Decide which purpose each of these serves. Visit the Learning Matters website (**www.learningmatters.co. uk/nursing**) to acquaint yourself with Stewart's analytical essay and determine which purpose this is meant to fulfil.

1.   The attached case study describes the experiences of Avril, a 35-year-old woman with learning difficulties. She lives within a community home with five other residents. Read the account of Avril's relationship with Tony, another resident, and then critically discuss the challenges that arise in association with contraception here.

2. *Nurses are necessarily interpreters of healthcare policies.* With reference to a policy of your own choosing, critically discuss whether you support this statement. Remember to back up your points with reference to the literature and/or observations from practice.

3. As part of a new initiative to engage the public in strategic healthcare planning, four ex-patients have become consultants to your nursing team. How will you work with them to enhance the services delivered to patients? Make sure that you refer to theories of leadership and change agency taught during your course.

Our reflections on this activity are given at the end of the chapter.

The case and the position taken

Having established the purpose of the forthcoming essay (what the question asks), our next job is to determine what position we take, and what case will be considered. The two are not necessarily the same. A case might be stated at the start of the essay and you are asked to examine it. You present questions and arguments that explain your position. In other instances, you make the opening case in the essay and back this up with arguments. Under examination conditions, being clear about the case and position is critical. However, we are often so keen to make best use of the time available that we set to, writing down points that are confused. We seem unsure about the case, and indecisive about our position. Yet we know that, by the end of the essay, our position has to be very clear. For example, relating to Activity 8.1, we might decide that we support the statement in (2) about nurses interpreting policy, but with certain caveats. There are some restrictions, because nurses must simultaneously apply several policies and each demands priority attention. So, you might support the case that nurses interpret policy, but your position is a qualified one.

Stewart confided to us that he didn't always clarify his position before writing essays. Certainly, his early exam work was 'position-confused', unlike the essay shared on the Learning Matters website. This was because he was fearful that the position he took would not seem the right one. He feared that examiners might judge him negatively if *his* perspective did not mirror theirs. He 'fudged matters', trying to write an answer that he hoped might please the examiner.

Reflect now on whether this worry has affected you too. Is it as important a problem as not knowing what your position is in the first place?

We share some thoughts on this at the end of the chapter.

Establishing your position is important. This is because it will determine what arguments you make within the essay and what evidence you draw on. Some positions require a great deal of evidence to support them, reflecting the complexity and ambiguities of nursing care. If we continue with the above example for a moment, we would need to identify circumstances where:

- we definitely should interpret the chosen policy;
- there is more limited scope to interpret the policy;
- factors combine to severely restrict our ability to interpret the policy.

On balance, if we support the case, the first group of these factors should pre-dominate. Showing that other factors intervene, though, and that there are caveats to consider, demonstrates that our judgement is not a rash one. In an essay such as this, we might draw on evidence from the literature that is connected to local protocols and standard care pathways, as well as observations from practice and discussions with colleagues who have managed policy implementation in the past.

Activity 8.3   Critical thinking

What sort of brief answer plan might you use in an examination situation to help you prepare an answer that demonstrates clearly your position in response to a question? Jot down an idea or two, perhaps describing a plan that you use now.

Our suggested plan is given at the end of the chapter.

Arguments and evidence

We have already seen in Chapter 3 that an essay is composed of a series of sections (introduction, main text, conclusion), which are, in turn, made up of a sequence of paragraphs, within which we advance our arguments. Coherent essays have arguments that fit with the position being defended and they lead appropriately to the conclusion. We might arrange the essay in several ways, for example reviewing the alternative positions that might be adopted with regard to nurses' interpretation of healthcare policy, before revealing the position that evidence seems to support. Alternatively, our position may seem so strong that we state this at the outset, and then lead the reader through stepwise arguments that demonstrate its power.

It is disempowering to feel that the only arguments that can fairly be advanced in an essay are those that are supported within the literature. This appears to suggest that the only valid form of knowledge is that which has been published. In truth, a significant amount of evidence remains unpublished and this includes some research findings, audits of practice and observations made in practice. There are different sorts of evidence and they make different contributions to a case (Pearson et al., 2007). Before you can couple evidence with your chosen arguments, though, you need to ascertain how powerful the evidence is and whether it clearly supports the point that you wish to make. A poorly selected piece of evidence can undermine your essay.

Activity 8.4   Critical thinking

Look at the following examples of evidence coupled with arguments that you might include within an essay on interpreting healthcare policy. Determine whether you think the evidence supports the chosen argument. Then decide which one of the

---

---

following examples of evidence/argument pairings seems too unconvincing to include in an essay. Finally, take a look at our reflections at the end of the chapter and return to Stewart's essay online to examine how he combines arguments and evidence to demonstrate his ability to reason.

1. **The argument**: Nurses are confident enough to examine policies critically, blending these with care philosophy to produce care that is workable and remains within the spirit of practice.
    The evidence: A conference paper presented by two nurse philosophers arguing that nurses have improved as discerning and articulate practitioners, and are able to determine what is beneficial, realisable and effective. The nurse philosophers report their grounded theory research, which included interviews with, and observations of, nurses in practice.
2. **The argument**: Nurses have been successful in advancing some areas of the chosen policy and delaying others, reflecting local circumstances and needs.
    The evidence: The International Council of Nurses has presented a series of findings on the role of the nurse as change agent.
3. **The argument**: There are standard care pathways that constrain healthcare professions, limiting the choices that practitioners can make.
    The evidence: Two standard care pathways in operation in local clinical areas are cited as examples of situations where practitioners sometimes express their frustration.

Our reflections are given at the end of the chapter.

Deciding which arguments and evidence make it into your essay is critical. You may have previously encountered essay feedback where the tutor has told you that your account was 'too superficial'. You are likely to be guilty of this if you try to include too many arguments and pieces of evidence. Evidence needs to be introduced and *you* need to make points about it. The exasperated assessor might observe, 'You seem to record everyone else's opinion, but not to synthesise these or to arrive at a perspective of your own!' Fewer arguments, then, and being more selective about what evidence you use to support them, will often stand your work in good stead.

Which of the following two short paragraphs seems the more developed, linking arguments and evidence together? The better of the two came from an essay with six key arguments, while the weaker one came from an essay with fourteen arguments.

1. Few would doubt that healthcare teams need to work corporately to achieve goals that have patients' welfare at heart, but there are reservations too. Nurses may wonder whether the organisation is more concerned with its own reputation, than with attending flexibly to the needs of the individual

> patient. Meeting targets for the many may limit what can be delivered to the individual. Trained as an advocate of patients, this leaves the nurse in a quandary: 'How will I individualise care when the organisation must attend to the masses?' Kirpal (2004) describes this as a challenge. Nurses see patients as clients and yet policy dictates that they work to corporate goals. Daily compromises then have to be reached by the nurse, sometimes contributing to what the organisation delivers on, and sometimes attending to the patient needs of the moment.
>
> 2. There is ample evidence that staff are deeply concerned to ensure that policy works well in practice. Moody (2004) describes work to arrange ethical hospital discharge for patients and McDonald et al. (2010) report on breastfeeding rates achieved by mothers. In practice, I have witnessed situations where nurses confer to determine when the policy will be applied in its pure sense and when it will be bent to suit a situation. Nurses sometimes search for other policies that they can refer to when explaining why the first has not been delivered in full. For example, policies promoting rapid patient discharge might be balanced by those associated with risk management and effective liaison with community teams. Nurses think hard about such things.
>
> *We give our verdict at the end of the chapter.*

Speculating successfully

Something that students find very difficult to achieve within an essay is speculation. If arguments are founded upon evidence, and evidence is contradictory or even absent, how do we proceed? We are left to rehearse what could be happening or what might be done next. We need to identify what can be suggested, whether that is within the literature or as part of clinical experience. We also need to imagine the future, how services might change, what patient needs could be, and how we might work better with relatives.

To speculate with confidence we need to use terms that signal to the reader that we have moved into speculative mode. We no longer argue something, or describe it, and we no longer claim it as fact – we speculate about it. If we signal these matters clearly and then write in a measured way about the subject (i.e., without stating what we think is 'obvious' or 'self-evident', or what 'naturally follows'), we will be taking the reader along with us, reasoning at our side.

The following words or short phrases all signal that we are speculating.

- **Notionally**: This suggests that we are considering an embryonic idea – one still in development. At this stage the idea is still a possibility, for example: 'Notionally, nurses do more to interpret policies than they realise. Even simple care involves interpreting what equals quality.'
- **Arguably**: This is used to suggest that the point is sufficiently clear and coherent to constitute an argument, but it is one we are still considering, for example: 'Nurses' frustration with policy is arguably to do with constraints on professional freedom. Nurses object to too many limits being set on their clinical decision making.'

- **We might speculate**: This is a very tentative way of putting things, suggesting an area of enquiry or a line of reasoning, for example: 'We might speculate that, while standard care plans save nurses' time, they also limit thinking. Where might I write about these concerns? There doesn't seem to be a box for that!'
- **A number of possibilities present**: This sets out possible explanations, for example: 'A number of possibilities present: first, that colleagues insist on writing their own policies; second, that they form alliances with the policy makers; and, third, that they lament change and continue to complain.'
- **It would be possible to suggest**: This hints that what is written about next has some credibility, for example: 'It would be possible to suggest that nurses are shaping the policies that matter – those that determine the experience of care.'
- **Conceivably**: This suggests something that could be considered, but might not be the easiest explanation, for example: 'Conceivably, nurse entrepreneurs are those who see policy as a lever. They use it to achieve desirable ends.'

Activity 8.6   *Reflection*

Look back over some past essays, and note whether you used any of the above words or phrases to indicate that you were speculating. Did you use the words in the right way? What happens if you use them too frequently in an essay?

We offer some ideas at the end of the chapter.

Reaching successful conclusions

A large majority of analytical essays written by students describe what has gone before within the essay, but without necessarily demonstrating a conclusion. To use a simple analogy, we describe a journey made (we spent three hours on the train). What is usually required within an analytical essay is to determine the significance of that journey. We can illustrate this by referring to the three purposes of analytical essays described earlier.

- The journey was arduous, took us longer than expected and prompted us to reconsider the advantages of using public transport in the future (evaluative).
- There remain opportunities to improve upon the journey, at least with regard to the time taken. Weekday public transport schedules are better (strategic).
- Travelling by public transport had the advantage of reducing our carbon footprint. Had we driven there, the environmental penalty would have been higher (philosophical).

A successful conclusion then must capture the account of what has been written so far (the journey), but must also include a deduction. We have to make clear what matters seem settled and what remain open at the end of the essay. Contrary to what some students think, it is not always true that we have to have 'nailed our colours to the mast', either adopting or rejecting the case. We do, however, have to have clarified our position.

In the following example of a concluding paragraph relating to the essay on policy interpretation, there is a clear indication of the author's resting position at the end. Notice how the author refers back to the case that has already been introduced at the start of the essay:

At the start of this paper, I introduced the case that nurses do interpret policies, but cautioned that their success in this is affected by factors that limit their freedom to proceed at will. The paper has noted that pressure of time and the need to serve a public, as well as individual patients, to work effectively in teams and to attend to employer agendas, all help determine the extent to which the nurse interprets policy. My chosen policy (rehabilitation) espouses a philosophy of cooperation and consultation. It remains an optimistic policy, at least where relatives' expectations are high and where the nurse must compromise, sharing care between patients. Nurses might wish to interpret this policy as an opportunity to deliver individualised care, but they don't always have the scope to proceed in that way. Instead, the need to ration their expertise and attention serves to contain just how much consultation they engage in.

In this conclusion, the journey is summed up quickly in the sentence describing what limits nurses' opportunities to interpret policy. The telling point arrives at the end, where it is explained that the nurse might wish to interpret policy in a particular way (as individualised care), but that care is necessarily rationed. The nurse does a little for the many and not as much as might be wished for the few. The author defends his or her opening case.

Activity 8.7   *Team working*

It is possible to practise the formulation of conclusions as part of a conversation with your colleagues. Working with three others, have the first colleague select a subject for the imaginary essay. The second should then briefly describe the case to be made there, and the third should summarise what the conclusion is (the case might or might not be supported). The fourth colleague should then be charged with determining whether the conclusion sounded convincing. Take it in turns to play different roles, choosing another essay subject, case and conclusion, and allowing all to practise their judgements.

As this activity is based on your own discussion, there is no answer at the end of the chapter.

Drafting the essay and checking its clarity

Students vary in their preferred ways of writing and editing. Having prepared an outline plan that signals the key sections of the paper, the arguments and evidence that will appear in each, the case that will be considered and the position adopted, some quickly set down a first draft. Students may have checked that they remain within the word counts they have allocated for each section, but they will leave the references, tables or quotations to be added later. The first goal for such students is to get work down on paper that captures their understanding of the subject and that represents their position regarding it. Other students move much more incrementally, carefully crafting each section and adding embellishments as they go. However you proceed, though, checking the clarity and coherence of what has been written there remains a responsibility.

We asked our four students about their essay drafting and reviewing processes.

Gina: 'If you write a "rough" draft of your essay in one sitting, you have the advantage that you don't pause to fret over doubts as you go. These will return to you later, though. Have I made this point clear, can I argue that, given what this article says?'

Fatima: 'I work with my plan, especially as regards the word allowance. If one section seems tight, and I need to include more words than I thought at first, I stop right then and ask whether I'm trying to include too much. It makes editing much easier.'

Raymet: 'I write first draft essays in the morning and then talk the content of my essay through with a friend. I explain what I am arguing. If they seem clear about my thoughts, even if they don't agree with my position, I feel encouraged.'

Stewart: 'Writing for me is private, but I always leave several days to complete an edit. My later essays have been better for that. I say to myself, "This isn't my essay, it's someone else's. I am going to pick it to pieces to see if it stands up."'

We agree with Gina that doubts can creep in as you write. It is just so easy to see multiple perspectives on a subject. Sometimes work grinds to a halt if you don't write a little more quickly and freely in the first instance. There is something to be said, then, for writing a first complete, but more rudimentary, draft. It probably captures your position most cleanly, provided that you have allocated enough thinking time before starting work.

Fatima's approach is much more 'sculpted'. The work proceeds in sections and each is 'got right' before the next is attempted. The approach does produce work that has well-balanced sections, each with a complement of words, arguments and evidence. It works well if you like to think in a stepwise fashion: 'This is what I must explain first; these are the context points. Next I must set out the case and suggest how my essay will examine that.' Students sometimes discover their position shifting a little as they write in this way. It is then necessary to check what is claimed in the introduction – do you still support that?

We especially support Raymet's strategy of summarising a first draft essay. Notice, though, that Raymet sticks to her guns once she has identified what her position will be. We think that this is commendable, *provided* you have heard and considered the questions and challenges posed by others. Your friend might not have read what you have, or attended the lectures that you did, so their position on a subject cannot be yours. Against that, naive questions and thoughtful challenges from reviewers are valuable, as you might well have missed something. To avoid charges of academic collusion and dishonesty, though, resist the temptation to ask them to edit your essay. This should remain your own work.

Stewart makes a good point when he describes how he distances himself from his own work at review stage. This is a fine example of evaluative critical thinking put to good use. The more you can imagine yourself as an editor, and less as the anxious author, the more likely you are to make the adjustments that help your work appear polished.

If you have left insufficient time to review work, or are preparing several papers in quick succession, essay editing can seem a bit of a chore. It is tempting to submit the work and hope. Time spent checking, however, is beneficial in several ways. You can:

- conduct the spelling, syntax and other presentational checks;
- ensure that the work answers the question or attends to the task set;
- assure yourself that a case has been made – one that is supported, rejected or seen as conditional within the conclusion;
- recount the arguments made and the evidence used ('Do they work together?').

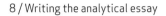

C H A P T E R   S U M M A R Y

Each individual essay is a work that operates in context, attending to the question or task set. Even though this is an academic work, it still expresses your preferred ways of working. You are the person who drafts the work and you write in a way that enables you to present scripts on time. There are, however, certain features of good analytical essay writing that show your critical thinking at work. You need to be very clear about the purpose of the essay and write in the appropriate way. Are you going to evaluate or philosophise, for example? You need to determine what case is being discussed and what position you take on it. In some instances, an examiner will set the case by making an assertion that you are invited to evaluate. In other instances, you select a case of your own – one that you will defend using arguments and evidence as your essay unfolds. Good analytical essay writing includes sufficient arguments and pieces of evidence to make a clear case. There is a balance struck between analytical writing (what I think) and descriptive writing (what I report). Where the debate remains open, and the best way forward is still to be discovered, you will make selective use of more speculative forms of writing. Conclusions are arranged in such a way that they do more than describe what has been discussed in the text. They indicate where your reasoning has led. All of this is improved where you allocate sufficient time to editing your own work.

Activities: brief outline answers and reflections

Activity 8.1: Critical thinking (pages 104–5)

1. This is a tricky one, isn't it? There are ethical/philosophical issues at stake here, surrounding human and reproductive rights, so the essay has a philosophical purpose. It is strategic too, though, as challenges in this instance seem to pose the question, 'What will you do next?' In these instances, the clues to what may be required often exist in the case study.
2. The purpose here is evaluative and the opening assertion, about nurses interpreting policy, makes this clear. Do you support this case?
3. The purpose here is strategic. The essay requires you to write about how you might involve lay consultants in the business of care delivery.

Activity 8.2: Reflection (page 105)

Some years ago, one of the authors of this book, Bob Price, conducted an informal audit of what consistently seemed to be associated with those essays that achieved better than average grades (A and B). He concluded that it was the clarity of the author's position with regard to the subject under discussion. However anxious learners were, they had trusted the system and staked a considered case for what was best, defensible or professional.

Activity 8.3: Critical thinking (page 106)

One that we have found workable is as follows.

- Essay purpose: what is asked of me?
- Case made: mine or the examiner's (name it)?
- My position: for or against the case, caveats noted.

- Section 1: introduction and signposting.
- Section 2: main body.
- Key arguments and paired evidence (argument 1, evidence; argument 2, evidence; etc.).
- Section 3: conclusions.

Activity 8.4: Critical thinking (pages 106–7)

1. The evidence here consists of research findings, but findings that might not have been published within the press. Research evidence is often thought of as more important than other forms, and in this case we would have felt more confident about it if the conference paper had to pass a peer review process before it was accepted. There seems to be a close connection made here to the argument that has to be supported.
2. Here, the evidence consists of something published by an august international body and one that, on this occasion, discusses change agency. Quite abstract points are perhaps made about nurses' change agency work, and it is not certain that there is a clear connection to the policy interpretation under question (there are many forms of change). This, then, would be the argument/evidence pairing that we might sacrifice in a shortened essay.
3. The evidence here is experiential and refers to local standard care pathways. It is clearly authentic to practice, as it deals with the same environments where the policy is being interpreted. There seems a potentially good fit between evidence and argument here.

Activity 8.5: Decision making (pages 107–8)

We think that paragraph (1) is the better of the two. While only one source of evidence is included (the work of Kirpal, 2004), there is a more extensive analysis of what this means. Readers could explore from this whether they have experienced similar dilemmas in working with a policy. While paragraph (2) refers to more examples of evidence, none of these is explored in any depth or connected in a clear way to the argument. More is not necessarily better.

Activity 8.6: Reflection (page 109)

Excessive use of speculative terms suggests that you have not made up your mind about many things. This may be honest and open, but it is usually expected that, in at least some areas of a subject, the author of an essay can venture a firmer opinion.

Knowledge review

To help you to evaluate your own grasp of the subject matter of this chapter, complete the following sentences.

1. My position in an essay is not necessarily the same as the case discussed and this is because . . .
2. Descriptive or superficial writing happens within an analytical essay when . . .
3. There are three purposes of analytical essays discussed within this chapter, and these are . . .
4. I can signal where I am speculating by using the following words or phrases . . .

Further reading

Gimenez, J (2007) *Writing for Nursing and Midwifery Students*. Basingstoke: Palgrave Macmillan.
This is an accessible textbook suitable for nurses on pre- and post-registration courses. It illustrates a wide range of writing forms, although connections to forms of thinking are not so well developed.

Greetham, B (2008) *How to Write Better Essays*, 2nd edition. Basingstoke: Palgrave Macmillan.
While this text is not written specifically for nurses, we think you will find it an accessible work and one that takes you through the essay planning process. There is a strong emphasis on personal organisation and preparation, as is common within such textbooks.

Useful website

www.lboro.ac.uk/library/skills/essay.html
Know-How: Essay writing, Loughborough University Library
Each university provides its own guide to essay writing, so you should seek out yours, especially with regard to conventions on referencing, which can vary between institutes. This site, however, is clear, accessible and provides a useful aide-memoire on the meaning of common question terms that you will encounter.

Chapter 9

Writing the reflective essay

NMC Standards for Pre-registration Nursing Education (2010)

This chapter will address the following competencies.

Domain: Professional values

8. All nurses must practise independently, recognising the limits of their competence and knowledge. They must reflect on these limits and seek advice from, or refer to, other professionals where necessary.

Domain: Leadership, management and team working

4. All nurses must be self-aware and recognise how their own values, principles and assumptions may affect their practice. They must maintain their own personal and professional development, learning from experience, through supervision, feedback, reflection and evaluation.

Chapter aims

By the end of this chapter you will be able to:

*   identify the important tasks to be attended to when writing the reflective essay;
*   discuss the functions of the reflective essay and how this affects its construction;
*   explain clearly the purpose of reflective essays;
*   demonstrate insights into the reporting of events, feelings, perceptions, perspectives, interpretations, conclusions and planned next actions associated with reflection;
*   utilise a chosen reflective framework in ways that help you to demonstrate your learning more clearly;
*   constructively criticise essay construction, using the case study example provided on the Learning Matters website.

Introduction

It is in the nature of nursing that we need to reflect and to be able to write reflectively. Nurses deal with human experience – that concerning health and illness, that linked to diagnosis and prognosis, and that attendant on difficult healthcare decisions. There are sometimes no trite 'right solutions' in healthcare, only best reasoned and argued courses of action, and these are founded to a significant extent upon reflection. It is because nurses need to access their experience, and that of others, in a clear and consistent way, and because we need to understand the process of reviewing and evaluating experience, that reflection and reflective writing are so important.

Reflection is also important if we are to manage successfully the stresses of nursing care. Our work is demanding, especially where we have discovered that we believe different things from other people, who may define care differently, value different goals and count other things as dignified and desirable. Our nursing work sometimes exposes us to conflict, disagreement and debate, so it is vital that we are able to make sense of such events if we are to continue caring in an open and sensitive way. We need to be aware of what we believe, value and espouse; we need to respect the beliefs of others, if we are to practise well (Seedhouse, 2009). Reflection, then, is important to our well-being, and to the preservation of a professional purpose in what we do.

In this chapter, we examine a series of key tasks associated with the business of writing reflectively – those linked to reflective writing coursework. Understanding these tasks will help you to write in ways that seem clearer and more coherent to others. Next, we give consideration to the reflective frameworks that you might be invited to use within your coursework. These vary by college and course, but certain principles are common to such frameworks. They all ask you to attend to feelings, meanings and then actions. After that, we consider the principles of best reflective writing practice and draw your attention to Raymet's example of a reflective essay, which can be found on the Learning Matters website (**www.learningmatters.co.uk/ nursing**). Reflective writing poses a number of challenges and examining an example essay is a useful way of reviewing these.

Five key tasks of reflective writing

Irrespective of whether your reflective writing takes the form of a coursework essay, a report from clinical practice placement, a case study of care planned and delivered, or a review of clinical decisions made, there are a number of tasks that your work should attend to.

Representing enquiry

Reflection is a form of enquiry that sees you return to experience, delve into attitudes and values, or explore the possibilities of practice. As we have seen in Chapter 2, reflection may happen while you are in action (delivering care) or after action (when you take a retrospective view). In the first of these instances your reflections are more likely to be formative – less well developed and without the benefit of hindsight. You will need to show the reader how you are speculating about what is happening, something we touched on in Chapter 8. All reflective writing, however, needs to explain quickly the purpose and the process of the enquiry in which you are engaged. Setting up these explanations at the start of your written work will help the reader to review your work with greater insight and perhaps to be more appreciative of what you achieve there.

We asked Fatima and Gina to share with us some of the opening paragraphs they have written at the start of reflective essays. Then we asked them to summarise these into a clear purpose and process for each. Their summaries are provided below. Read each of these and then prepare brief notes on why working on such summaries might improve your reflective essay writing.

Fatima: 'The purpose of this essay is to explore the ways in which I negotiated care with a family supporting a dying patient. To that end, I arrange my reflections using a series of headings, those first associated with my assumptions and perceptions of care needs, those that I believed that the family held, and then the compromises that were sought as we tried to bring our expectations of care together.'

Gina: 'The purpose of this essay was to uncover some of the values, beliefs and aspirations that I hold with regard to holistic care. This work involved critical reflections regarding what each element of holistic care entails, and what my skills and work capacity could reasonably deliver on. My reflections conclude with a summary of the discrepancies that remain, between what I believe I should deliver and what I succeed in assisting patients with.'

We offer notes of our own at the end of this chapter.

Distinguishing between facts, perspectives and perceptions

Reflective writing deals with facts (e.g., the dosage of a drug taken), but it also deals regularly with perspectives and perceptions, and we need to show that we appreciate distinctions between these within our work. A perspective is something that sums up our position, values, aspirations and beliefs. For example, 'Care should be patient centred, working with the individual's needs' is an expression of a perspective. It is often used to describe what we think should be the case or what should happen. A perception, though, is much more fragile than this and describes the impressions that we take from incomplete or fragmentary experience. 'Mrs Jones was confused by the news; she seemed to search for words to express all the worries that suddenly arose inside her' is an example of a perception. We have no direct proof of what Mrs Jones felt, as she has not told us, but we infer that her behaviour and her hesitant words were indicative of anxiety.

Much of what we reflect upon in essays revolves around these three things: facts, perceptions and perspectives. A number of mistakes are easily possible as we draft our work.

- We may allow our perspective to dominate how we imagine others think or feel (they must be like me, believe what I believe, value what I value).
- We may infer perspectives held by others based on quite limited perceptions of what they do or say (we, as it were, fill in the gaps, explaining to ourselves why others act as they do).
- We may build a perspective on a subject based on a series of perceptions, each of which is reasonable in and of itself, but which collectively become more suspect as we string these together. We overextend our critical reflection, claiming more than seems reasonable.

- We muddle perception and fact, writing about perceptions *as* fact. In this instance, we forget how transient or tentative our impressions are, and we allow ourselves to feel more sure about something than is justified.

To write successfully it is necessary to be clear about whether you are writing about a fact, a perspective or a perception. In many of the best reflective essays, nurses write about competing perspectives or perceptions. They recount their first impressions of a situation, describe how this changes, and speculate about the perceptions that others may have regarding the situation. Rather than close that debate, arguing that this or that is therefore the case, they acknowledge that the situation remains ambiguous and that further interpretation is needed. Here is a successful example of that from Gina's work on holistic care:

> *Spiritual care was challenging for me, as I typically associated it with religious belief and especially my religious beliefs. So my default perspective was that, to talk about spiritual care, was to talk about how others live their religious convictions. It seemed apparent, though, that other people, including those who were not overtly religious, also had a sense of the spiritual. This appeared to be associated with that which was aesthetic, beautiful, meaningful, especially as regards good living in its different guises. I discovered that it was about that which made people feel dignified and good about themselves, about that which made them more than a role, someone with a purpose as well as a function in society. It was about what they described as 'me'.*

Demonstrating insight

In many instances reflective writing also requires that you take a risk and that you share with the reader some insights into your beliefs, ways of thinking and operating. At best, these insights demonstrate your quizzical attitude towards what you do or believe. It can feel uncomfortable to write in this way, especially if you fear that the examiner will condemn you for what we haven't achieved. In a healthcare culture that expects consistency and excellence, perhaps beyond human or system capacity, it is more difficult to confide things about what seemed imperfect within yourself and remained open to improvement or revision.

To help you share insights in this way, it is worth checking with your tutor in advance that the essay is being assessed as evidence of continued learning and professional growth. Well-written assignment briefs should make this apparent from the outset, although you should note caveats about professional standards. To confide that you have behaved in an unprofessional or illegal manner may still mean that the work triggers some form of sanction. The reflective essay is not a confessional that absolves you of all guilt for acts that have been dangerous or demeaning for patients.

Activity 9.2   *Reflection*

Pause now to write a short passage of reflective work in which you express doubts about your own reasoning or decision making. Alternatively, use the passage to explore what might be incomplete or incoherent in your care philosophy, much as Gina does in Activity 9.1 above. Try to determine where you have thought too narrowly, a little naively or without reference to some important information.

When you have prepared this, turn to the example that we share at the end of this chapter and review our brief notes on what seems successful in such writing.

Respecting others

When writing reflectively, we run the risk that we express prejudices, opinions and attitudes that demonstrate a disregard for the rights and dignity of others. This is not simply a matter of political correctness. While you are advised in reflective essays or case studies to create pseudonyms for others discussed within your answer (protecting their identity), expressing prejudicial and unsubstantiated views about them is still likely to prompt criticism of your work. Nurses respect and support the dignity of others (Seedhouse, 2000). It is necessary, then, to write circumspectly and to consider carefully whether expressed attitudes might signal a disregard for patients or colleagues, cause offence to the reader, or suggest that we might practise in ways that could be detrimental to nursing. This requirement relates not only to those of a different gender, age, colour, culture, religious background or sexual identity from your own, but to any with whom you have professional working relationships. Check, therefore, that what you include in your reflection demonstrates a respect for others. By all means acknowledge difference – the diversity of human experience and need, but don't assume that your own perspectives on matters are superior.

Illustrating learning

Your reflective essay has one further function and that is to demonstrate your learning. If you write in a static way, about an unquestioned perspective or perceptions that seem set in stone, you are unlikely to have attended to the last of the five tasks – the illustration of learning. Good reflective writing takes the reader on a journey, from that which is shared at the start of the essay to that which is shared at the end. In this regard, reflective writing stands in sharp contrast to other forms of academic writing. In the analytical essay, the student often creates a case and then defends that using a series of arguments within the main text (see Chapters 3 and 8). In reflective writing, however, the approach is revelatory. As the paragraphs and sections unfold, the reader gains a sense of your reasoning as it changes and grows. Figure 9.1 illustrates what we mean by this, using a flow chart and some of Gina's work on holistic practice.

Activity 9.3   *Critical thinking*

At the next opportunity, take a moment to revisit a piece of your own reflective writing and try to describe the movement in your thinking that you share there.

- Is there a deepening of your appreciation of the complexity of healthcare?
- Do you understand something new about the diversity of need?
- Do you demonstrate a process of debate underway as you consider what you encounter?

In some past essays, there may be little or no movement in your thinking and you could usefully consider what would show you learning as you wrote. In others, the movement may be inconsistent. In one passage you move towards one perspective and in another passage towards a different one. The reader cannot easily determine what you are concluding about your experiences.

- Does this suggest something important to you as regards reflecting before you write?

We share brief remarks on this last point at the end of the chapter.

Figure 9.1: Reflecting and learning.

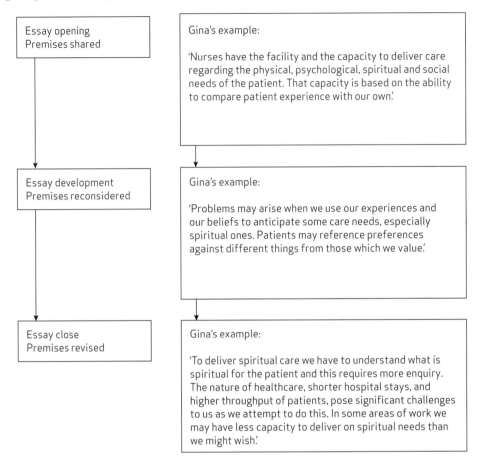

Using reflective frameworks

Many students learn the process of reflective writing using one or other of the reflective practice frameworks. Ashby (2006) notes that a key benefit of using reflective frameworks or models is that we learn the discipline of seeing experiences from different perspectives. We 'frame' experiences in different ways and are then able (with others) to discuss the perspectives that we develop, adopt or abandon en route. Among the reflective frameworks commonly used within nursing courses are those proposed by Gibbs (1988) and Johns (1995). In the Gibbs framework, we are encouraged to do the following.

1. **Clearly describe the situation**. Without premature judgement, state what happened, or what we understand to be factual.
2. **Explore our feelings**. Feelings are often a filter through which we read events. Does this experience represent a threat, an accolade, a challenge or affirmation of what we do? Do feelings help me understand what was challenging, difficult, delightful or encouraging here?
3. **Evaluate the experience**. Was this was positive, negative, confusing or ambiguous?
4. **Reflect**. Make sense of the experience. Do we have a chance to learn here, and to confirm what counts as excellent? Is this something that helps me to

understand a wider range of healthcare needs, or the consequences of action or inaction?

5. **Conclude**. What we take away from this? Can these lessons be applied elsewhere?
6. **Act**. What we might do differently in the future?

Johns' model of structured reflection draws upon Carper's different ways of knowing in nursing (Carper, 2004). We not only reference our insights against the events as they unfolded, but against different ways of thinking.

- **Aesthetic knowing** refers to values within nursing and about care. It attends to the style or manner in which care is delivered – what seems most valuable in what is being done. We are prompted to ask ourselves questions about what we were trying to achieve, why we responded as we did in this situation, and what we think the consequences of our stance or action might be for others. We are challenged to determine what we think other people were feeling and to explain how we know this.
- **Personal knowing** directs the nurse to a review of his or her own feelings, for example what influenced whether care seemed satisfactory, unsettling or challenging.
- **Ethical knowing** challenges us to review the beliefs that guide our work. Will we base our work on some inalienable rights of the patient, or instead consider what are the most likely and beneficial outcomes of what we do or don't do?
- **Empirical knowing** attends to what knowledge underpinned our reasoning and actions. It is worth considering here whether empirics refers solely to research evidence, and what can be established as fact, or whether it also includes theories as well. In most instances, nurses have tended to clump all of these things together under empirical knowing, arguing that there seems no other place to record points about theoretical knowledge.
- **Reflexive knowing** (seeing ourselves as actors within the experience – figures that influence events) prompts us to think back over past experiences and to relate our actions today with those in the past, to determine what options were open to us here and may be so in the future.

At their best, reflective frameworks assist us to showcase our learning. As we consider matters such as the aesthetics of care, review the ways in which beliefs and feelings shaped what we did, we demonstrate both insight and change. At the end of the essay we can state what we might do differently in the future, because we can articulate what experience has taught us in the past. Writing using the reflective frameworks, however, requires a little thought. We commend the following.

- Start by making a series of points that you wish to write about and decide under which framework heading these will appear (otherwise you might make the same point in more than one place). If the point has several different dimensions, for example both aesthetic and knowledge elements, be clear how you are discussing the point differently in each place.
- If you find that there are no points for some framework headings, decide whether this matters. In the Johns framework, for example, it is not automatic that all experiences will necessarily have an ethical dimension. If you use the Gibbs framework, though, you should be able to complete all stages 1–6 in the reflective process.
- Determine what opportunities exist to discuss your reflections and when these occur. If you are writing a formative piece of work – one that is not assessed on a

pass or fail basis, especially if there is an opportunity as a group to discuss reflections after each has been presented, there is benefit in writing freely and deliberating more deeply afterwards in the company of others. You are able to refine your reflection and the essay becomes a 'work in progress'. If the work is submitted for assessment purposes, it is necessary to deliberate fully on your reflections at the time of essay construction.

- Don't be afraid to discuss key concepts with your tutor. In reflective writing, clarity in the use of concepts and their consistent use in the essay are important. For example, are you confident in your understanding of what counts as aesthetic?

Activity 9.4	Critical thinking

Look at the following points made by students and determine which sort of knowing they refer to: aesthetic, personal, ethical, empirical or reflexive. Add a note explaining why.

1. I felt a dilemma immediately: should I support the patient or her well-meaning daughter? The patient reasoned inconsistently as a result of her dementia, while her daughter seemed to have (on the face of it) a better understanding of what care a nursing home might offer. The mother wanted independence at all costs, even if more risk was involved. But the daughter had her own motives; she had been caring for her mother a long time.

2. The disappointment that I felt, while delivering care to older people for the first time, surprised me. I felt disbelief and disillusionment, and all because the sheer energy and resources required to support patients really well seemed beyond the facilities currently available.

3. The underpinning rationale for the use of memory boxes with older people seemed well established. Not only did memory boxes help older people to take stock of their past, they also facilitated conversation between patients. They were stimulating and interesting, and enabled younger people, nurses and visitors to learn about and respect the past lives of the patients on the ward.

4. It seemed important to me to establish just what the patient understood about risk and, as far as was possible, to help her make a decision about those risks that seemed acceptable and those that were not. What supports dignity is making choices, even if sometimes they are not necessarily the best choices. It seemed unrealistic to try to insulate the patient against all risks. My role was to help her manage those that were most likely to arise, and especially those that had significant implications for her.

5. If experience was teaching me anything, it has been about artful compromise, which still expresses my nursing values clearly, but which also demonstrates my adaptability, imagination and problem solving. This incident could be reviewed in terms of ideals, but my reflections above all show the need to search for solutions that enable the majority to feel that progress is being made. In the future, as today, it is necessary to search for solutions that fit with the requirements in hand. There is no neat formula to determine what quality care is comprised of.

Compare your answer with ours at the end of the chapter.

Identifying best practice in reflective writing

In this penultimate section, we draw your attention to Raymet's example essay, which is available on the Learning Matters website (**www.learningmatters.co.uk/nursing**), and identify some best practice principles in the different sections of a reflective essay. Raymet writes reflectively, using the Gibbs framework outlined above, but many of the points we share here, about objectivity and feelings for example, hold good in other reflective essays too.

Describing the situation

The description of the situation is usually presented either within an extended introduction, or as the second section of the essay. In Raymet's case, she uses the introduction to signal her intention to reflect on issues relating to the assessment of pain and to indicate how the rest of the essay is set out (a signpost paragraph).

When describing a situation it is important to do the following.

- Include sufficient information to help the reader understand your subsequent reflections (Raymet alerts us to some ambiguities in the way Mrs Drew has reported her pain in the past. This is an important context as she tries to read this patient's concerns now).
- Avoid offering excess, irrelevant information. It is possible to overload the reader with contextual information, so that it is then difficult for them to understand what you have focused on. Staffing levels in Raymet's work setting, for example, would probably not be of central importance to her reflection.
- Report only what has happened and not (at this stage) your interpretation of the same. It is useful here to think of yourself as a police officer, who dispassionately records events without surmising motives or agendas. To this end, your writing should focus on observed behaviour. Raymet does this well in her essay, but she confided to us that it was only after redrafting this section two or three times. The urge to interpret can be strong!

Exploring feelings

It is *your* feelings that should be the primary focus here. Any feelings that you write about with regard to others will necessarily be based on perceptions or feelings that others have reported to you. The purpose of the reflective essay is not to recount all the perceived feelings within any one situation, but to understand your own emotions as you deliver care. The purpose of reviewing your feelings is to consider these as a filter – as an influence upon how you reason about care. Strong emotions can result in us foreclosing on our interpretations of events. The patient was *obviously* this, the staff *clearly* intended that – we prematurely limit what experience can teach us and may subsequently act in a less thoughtful way. Mixed emotions can serve to stifle decisions, and to produce courses of action that seem inconsistent or incoherent.

Activity 9.2 has already practised you in an introspective form of writing, but, within this section of the essay, that needs to be applied to your own feelings. Your emotions might be observed:

- as alarming or surprising (perhaps you were startled by the strength of your emotions);
- as difficult to access or interpret (your feelings shifted and changed);
- as going counter to rational reasoning (I expected this, but experienced that);

- as challenging your assumptions (something that Gina has already shared with us in this chapter);
- as adding to your appreciation of why care is exhilarating, exciting and challenging.

It may be tempting to analyse your feelings critically in some depth within this section, but we recommend that you reserve the deeper analysis for the next two sections. At this stage it is sufficient to acknowledge the feelings that can influence your interpretation of events and shape your approach to care.

Evaluating the experience

Your evaluation of the experience involves making some measured judgements. The events discussed, the decisions made and the actions chosen may be more or less successful, more or less appropriate, more or less sensitive and patient centred. They may betoken well-informed action or best action available, given the information to hand. They will usually entail a return to the feelings reported in the last section (did these lead us to specific interpretations?). In most instances, we can evaluate the experience as an opportunity for learning, and as something that can teach us new ways of thinking or working. But this observation only works well in an essay if we can express what was instructive about the experience. Raymet's case study essay (on the Learning Matters website) is well developed in this regard; she is able to capture the events succinctly and to suggest what they represent. In this case, that is an opportunity to question more deeply the theory of pain assessment, especially that pertaining to the measurement of pain.

Reflecting

The evaluation that you report in the preceding section of the essay is, in many regards, a first evaluation – an initial considered impression. There is scope within the section on reflecting to extend learning a good deal further. In a reflective essay on pain assessment this might take several forms, for example:

- raising questions about how we use pain assessment tools;
- speculating about what insights into patient accounts of symptoms might teach us in other settings;
- highlighting what is missing or misconceived within our assessment approach.

As word allowances constrain all essays, you will need to be circumspect about how widely you range when discussing the implications of what you have heard, seen and done. It is usually better to reflect on a few select things well and convincingly, rather than to skate over a large number of points in a more superficial way. Remember, the purpose of the reflective essay is to demonstrate your learning. To this end, you need sufficient words to show movement in your thinking of the kind already summarised in Figure 9.1.

Concluding

Some students struggle to make clear distinctions between reflections and conclusions. They write about their reflections (what we might think of as musings or speculations) as though they were also conclusions. The problem is rather akin to reporting a mathematical equation and offering the answer, without demonstrating how you arrived at it. Your conclusions should sum up your reflections and suggest where (for now) your reflections rest. It is not necessarily the case that you have discovered 'the solution', merely that you report a stage of thought – where you stand today. Tomorrow, further learning may be possible or necessary.

As in other sorts of essays, it is possible to write conclusions that overstate what you have discovered, and that overextend what can reasonably be claimed from your reflections so far. It is better to represent learning today, so far, rather than to claim insights that have no basis in reflection to date. While nurses are eager to solve problems, and to make circumstances better for patients, one of the benefits of reflection is that it teaches you about your limitations too.

Signalling future action

Sometimes it is possible to signal a future course of action – a new way forward – and sometimes it is not. There will be occasions when the best you can do is to indicate issues that remain unresolved. As with conclusions, it is wise not to overstate these, especially where they presume the provision of resources and how others, as well as ourselves, will behave in future. Remember, yours is a personal and a professional reflection. It is based on your experience and evaluation of events. Your conclusions are not necessarily shared by others, so consultation and collaboration are usually important at this future action stage. Assessors are usually more than content to reward accounts of how *you* will think differently, and approach care situations more sensitively and thoughtfully – important professional attributes of the nurse.

C H A P T E R   S U M M A R Y

Reflective writing requires just as much discipline as other forms of academic work, but in this instance attends to the interpretation of events and the representation of your learning, conclusions and planned next actions. You demonstrate to the reader the sense that you have made of experience. Reflective writing will be clearer, more effective and more convincing if you are clear about the purpose of a given essay, if you use reflective frameworks consistently and transparently, and if you arrange your points under the relevant section headings of the work. You may feel that you have a natural aptitude for reflection and writing about experience. Alternatively, you may feel happier writing in other ways. Reflective writing, though, is an important discipline for nurses.

Activities: brief outline answers and reflections

Activity 9.1: Communication (page 117)

Summaries such as these aid your writing because they highlight what you will reflect on and how that reflection will be set out within the body of your essay. While we might reflect generally upon experiences ('That was a terrible train journey'), it is always more productive and educational to link reflection to a purpose ('The train journey was long, but when we compare this with the cost of travel by air and the time it would take by road . . .'). Reflection in nursing is not simply a norm or a duty, it has a purpose, and this is to enhance your reasoning and care planning abilities. So purpose and process are important. The more you understand what you are doing and why, the more coherent your thinking is likely to be.

Activity 9.2: Reflection (page 118)

Here is my reflective paragraph, which you believe demonstrates a measured and critical evaluation of what was discovered during a community placement. The passage relates to giving advice on nutrition to patients, some of whom don't have the resources to which we might be accustomed.

> *It seems possible to treat the 'well-balanced diet' as a mantra that I was all too ready to chant with patients: 'Do this, eat that and you will remain healthy.' I was repeating a formula and not stopping to examine the implications of what I said. Neville, an elderly gentleman I visited within an inner-city borough, brought me up short: 'Look lass, can you tell me what the cost is of a Sunday joint, a mix of fresh vegetables and some fruit out of season?' I shook my head; I couldn't. My comfortable lifestyle had never demanded that I pause to consider such things. 'Well,' he continued, 'I can tell you that it's dearer than a packet of supermarket budget biscuits and less comforting than the bottle of stout I drink each night. Some of us exist on different things. Some of us either can't afford fresh fruit or else we prefer to sup something that gives us pleasure.' I felt mortified. I had offered Neville the textbook answer and he hadn't read my textbook. I wasn't thinking at all clearly or incisively and now I had irritated a patient who probably saw me as a middle-class busybody.*

Notice how I use quotes from the patient to capture the challenge encountered during placement. Notice, too, how I register shock at the patient's response: 'I felt mortified.' I move on to suppose how Neville might see me, reflecting on the lost opportunity to advise him on his diet in more sensitive ways. I don't condemn myself, but neither do I pull punches. I had assumed something about a patient, without sufficient information.

Activity 9.3: Critical thinking (page 119)

Our point here would be that reflective writing is both a process and a product. The very act of writing something down can trigger new insights. We learn as we write. In nursing courses, however, many such essays are products too – representations of your learning. They are assessed and graded. To that end, you should either roughly draft reflections where you can try out your insights before you prepare the essay, or else you should be prepared to go back and edit your work – not simply with regard to syntax and spelling, but with regard to arranging points that show how your thinking has changed.

Activity 9.4: Critical thinking (page 122)

1 = ethical

Reference to a 'dilemma' here should have alerted you to the fact that this is writing about ethics and the challenges that arise there. The nurse perceives the need to make a choice between patient and relative, but she could also select a third option, to mediate a compromise.

2 = personal

This writing concerns feelings, in this case disappointment. The disappointment is qualified with reference to expectations. This is not how she expected care to be in this setting.

3 = *empirical*

While this student doesn't refer to research and offer a reference here (she probably should have as regards the use of memory boxes!), this is certainly work concerned with empirical matters. She critically examines the memory boxes in use.

4 = *aesthetic*

This student is expressing a series of points about values – her values and the importance of patient choice. Our values form an important reference point when discussing the aesthetics of care.

5 = *reflexive*

This excerpt comes from an essay conclusion and is appropriately reflexive. The student is taking stock of their learning and the importance of searching for compromises.

Knowledge review

Answer the following questions. If you struggle with any of these, revisit the above text to help you consolidate your learning.

1. Why is it an advantage to have a clear purpose in mind when planning a reflective essay?
2. How can we distinguish between facts, perspectives and perceptions?
3. How can we demonstrate learning within a reflective essay?
4. What are the key advantages of using a reflective framework to present reflections on practice?
5. What is it important to remember when describing events, recording conclusions and summarising next actions within a reflective practice essay?

Further reading

Bulman, C and Schutz, S (eds) (2004) *Reflective Practice in Nursing: The growth of the professional practitioner*, 3rd edition. Oxford: Blackwell.
While this collection of essays deals with reflective practice more generally, there are excellent chapters on supporting reflection in others, and in the assessment and evaluation of reflective writing.

Buck, A, Sobiechowska, P and Winter, R (1999) *Professional Experience and the Investigative Imagination: The art of reflective writing*. London: Routledge.
What is especially exciting and stimulating about this book is the way it discusses reflective writing in storytelling terms. We tell stories to explain what happened, who we are, what we stand for . . .. Myths are an example of storytelling used to convey exceptional meanings and beliefs. Reading this book affords fresh insights into the process of reflecting and writing that we think are as relevant in healthcare today as yesterday.

Useful websites

www.brookes.ac.uk/services/upgrade/a-z/reflective_writing.html
This is the website of Oxford Brookes University and its student support services. While most universities post some advice on different ways of writing, this one is exceptionally

detailed and clear, providing guidance on the use of several different reflective frameworks, including those of Gibbs and Johns. The pdf examples of reflective writing are very welcome additions to the site.

www.rcgp.org.uk/default.aspx?page=5555
This is the website of the Royal College of General Practitioners and summarises the reflective writing workshops arranged there. It is valuable because it offers examples of GPs' reflective writing. It can be very instructive to see how other healthcare professionals write reflectively and to compare and contrast this with your personal or college approach.

Chapter 10

Building and using your portfolio of learning

NMC Standards for Pre-registration Nursing Education (2010)

This chapter will address the following competencies.

Domain: Professional values

7. All nurses must be responsible and accountable for keeping their knowledge and skills up to date through continuing professional development. They must aim to improve their performance and enhance the safety and quality of care through evaluation, supervision and appraisal.

Domain: Nursing practice and decision making

1. All nurses must use up-to-date knowledge and evidence to assess, plan, deliver and evaluate care, communicate findings, influence change and promote health and best practice.

Chapter aims

By the end of this chapter you will be able to:

*   discuss the best ways to set out a portfolio;
*   appreciate the advantages of building a portfolio;
*   identify the ways in which you are thinking critically as you compile and use your portfolio;
*   suggest ways in which individual reflections can be built on through the portfolio;
*   identify a range of circumstances under which drawing excerpts from your portfolio might enable you to make a case about either your development or your professionalism.

Introduction

Portfolios of learning, learning journals or logs, and personal professional profiles are used widely within higher education and the nursing profession beyond, to help nurses organise a coherent account of their achievements, enquiries and development. Unlike diaries, they combine hard evidence of experience (e.g., a practice placement record) with reflexive evidence of learning (e.g., a series of structured reflections on what has been discovered). Registered nurses are required as part of their post-registration education and practice (Prep) requirements to maintain a personal professional profile, which provides evidence of at least 35 hours' learning completed every three years (NMC, 2010a). While the term used to describe such records may vary slightly from setting to setting, the rationale remains the same. The portfolio exists to represent nurses' development over time, the areas that they have enquired into and what they have deduced or mastered there. The portfolio allows the nurse to make a case not only about what has been learned, but also why this is relevant to his or her practice and, in the case of students, how course learning outcomes have been met.

This chapter sets out guidance on the building and the use of a portfolio as part of your professional work as a nurse. It highlights the part that critical and reflective thinking play. You are encouraged to read this in conjunction with any course or university requirements relating to the format of the portfolio. For example, in some instances this will be a hard copy document that you carry with you to interviews and placements. In other situations it may be an electronic document or even a collection of documents, stored within your personal space on the course website. In building and presenting your portfolio it is necessary to remain mindful of the requirements set down by the university or professional organisation that reviews such work. The NMC, for example, sets out relatively short and simple requirements as regards the personal professional profile (NMC, 2010a, pp26–7). To meet update requirements, your profile entries should:

- state what you do (your role);
- date the entry (so that auditors can evaluate learning over time);
- describe the learning activity (e.g., completion of a reading programme, attendance at a study day);
- state the number of learning hours completed (this in practice is often an estimate, especially if learning comprises work-based informal learning);
- describe what the learning consisted of, and what insights you gained or understanding/skill you developed;
- summarise the outcome of the learning activity (e.g., what you can now do, how your attitudes have changed).

Portfolio building is not something that all nurses turn to eagerly. Unlike an artist who must show a portfolio of work to gain new commissions or exhibition opportunities month by month, registered nurses are only periodically required to illustrate their achievements. We are not all diary keepers or plan makers in the sense that portfolios facilitate. Nonetheless, the portfolio skills that you develop on your course will stand you in good stead later, not only to help you pass assessments, but also to make a best case regarding your credentials when you apply for a new job or promotion, or where you perhaps make an application to a postgraduate course. Portfolios of learning can sometimes enable you to claim accreditation for prior experiential learning, shortening the length of study that you need to do in subsequent courses, or gaining you entry into a course where you do not hold the best fit entry qualifications.

Choosing or designing a portfolio of your own

While some universities issue students with a formatted learning log that they are required to use, most allow the student carte blanche to develop one of their own, provided that it complies with certain requirements. At minimum this means that there is space for a record of experience and courses or modules completed (here you may keep a record of clinical placements, visits, projects or field trips conducted); a place where you reflect on what your experience, teaching or enquiry has taught you (this section usually requires that you relate your insights to course learning outcomes); and a space where you can write up your aims and strategies for further enquiry (this is the prospective part of the portfolio and provides a chance for you to demonstrate your strategic thinking). In theory, then, a portfolio can be successfully built using a loose-leaf folder and some dividing cards to enable you to create sections within your work. What is important is that, whatever format your portfolio takes, it should be:

- logically arranged and accessible (with sections and contents pages);
- consistently arranged (e.g., using standard sections, subsections and headings);
- well presented (avoiding spelling and syntax errors; communication is important in this area of nursing, as in all others);
- up to date and representative of your learning (records that peter out several months ago prompt questions about what you have done more recently).

For students who have access to an electronic learning space associated with their course, there are real advantages in keeping an electronic portfolio. The advantage of this format is that you can readily update or change your entries, building and representing evidence of achievement as you go along. The record is less static than if it was presented on a printed page, but remains open to printing whenever you need it. If you use this format, however, you need to be sure that it can be downloaded to your own computer after the course is completed, as several elements of this work may be relevant to your future career. It is necessary to check the university rules as regards the use and privacy terms relating to this record, and to respect any restrictions placed there on the nature of records that can be made.

Critical thinking and your portfolio

Portfolios consist of several different sorts of evidence that are arranged as a coherent whole to represent your learning. The way in which you order this evidence, relating one sort to another and linking all to your strategic plans, demonstrates a great deal about your ability to conceptualise (e.g., identifying problems and learning needs), to analyse (e.g., what seemed to be possible ways forward) and to strategise (e.g., selecting the right enquiries to make). A very simple arrangement for the portfolio could be as shown in Table 10.1.

Table 10.1: Possible simple portfolio layout.

Portfolio section	Design notes
Preliminary section, including your name, contact details, contents list and list of key reference sources (websites, telephone numbers, email addresses).	This is a precious document, so including your name and contact details is important were it to be lost. 'Lost' here can include computer crashes, so be sure to back up your portfolio files on a regular basis, storing these in a place beyond the computer itself. Your contents list needs to include sections and then a list of all entries in each. Be consistent in your approach as you will probably need to cross-reference material within the portfolio, for example entry one within your first section becomes 1.1 and so on. Adding an aide-memoire of the web addresses for key enquiry resources, and for those within the library and beyond is also helpful as they are to hand whenever you update your portfolio.
Section 1: Evidence of achievements, courses or learning, projects or field trips completed.	You need a section where you can include all the different sorts of evidence that testify to the experience that you have gained. Label each entry so that it corresponds to your contents list. Entries here may take different forms, and may include, for example, certificates of attendance or course completion, reference lists of reading programme papers reviewed, or copies of reports relating to clinical placements. Note, however, that this evidence does not in itself always demonstrate learning. Simply listing articles read doesn't tell us what you deduce from your reading. You will therefore need to either add short reflective annotations to some entries, or else cross-reference the entry in your next section, where you write up your reflections more extensively. Because your portfolio needs to remain a 'live and current document', it will be periodically necessary to replace some very old pieces of evidence with that which has superseded it. Were this not to be the case, you would have a portfolio in several volumes and with some early entries of only historical interest. Check with your tutor, though, before doing this on a course. Here evidence is not usually replaced until course end.

Table 10.1: Continued

Section 2: Evidence of reflection and debate, and the meanings that you ascribe to experience.	Each entry in this section is likely to be referenced against one or more course learning outcomes, and to utilise the reflective framework that you have chosen or that has been required by the college. If no such restrictions apply, you might consider using the entry headings recommended by the NMC (see above). Evidence here may relate to clinical experience, reflections upon workshop activities or seminars, debates that have arisen after a lecture, or observations made after shadowing a more experienced practitioner. Wherever experience offers a constructive learning opportunity there is scope to make an entry. Don't forget that reflections are not necessarily one to one – a reflection for each individual experience. Sometimes you will write reflections relating to a series of experiences. This is why a system of cross-referencing is important in your portfolio.
Section 3: Plans, future aims and learning strategies.	You might expect this section to appear at the front of the portfolio, but, as learning is incremental and plans are frequently revised, we suggest that it appears at the end. The wording of your entries here is important. Try to ensure that you are specific in what you set out to do (the aim), that you detail how you will achieve that aim (the method), that you note any anticipated resources that you will use (support), and that you set a realistic time-frame for completion of the work planned. If someone else will verify your learning, perhaps your personal tutor, make space for their signature in the paperwork. Resist the temptation to set out with grand plans, multiple aims and unrealistic time-frames. Identify fewer achievable aims and progress from there.

Of the four students whose learning we have reported in this book, Fatima was the most enthusiastic and well organised with regard to her portfolio of learning. We discussed with her the different ways in which her portfolio represented her critical thinking to others. Four things stood out.

- The number of connections made between entries within her portfolio. There were very clear connections made between plans and subsequent evidence of learning, and the cross-referencing enabled the reader to follow this. For example, section 2 entries cross-referenced the relevant section 3 plan and alerted the reader to any additional evidence of achievement within section 1.
- The discrimination shown as regards the number of entries made. Fatima's wasn't the biggest or heaviest portfolio submitted for assessment, but it was the best. She explained:

I knew from the start that I couldn't record every experience and reflection, it would be exhausting. As my portfolio grew the record would become ever more complex! For that reason I started jotting down rough notes on experiences and then writing up only those that stood the test of time, or else combining reflections on several incidents to demonstrate how I brought ideas together.

The portfolio is a working document, so some elements will remain work in rough, while others will become refined – they become part of the end product submitted for assessment.

- The focus of the entries made. These attended closely not only to the learning outcomes set within her course, but also to the different sorts of experience she was having. The examiners noted how differently she thought when supporting different groups of patients and working in different settings. She was clearly able to adapt her thinking to context and need.
- The way in which her plans evolved. There was clear evidence of Fatima's quest for knowledge, in her independent study as well as in what others taught or shared. Fatima noted:

I was quite tempted to dump some of my early plans from the portfolio, because they seemed naive. My tutor, though, helped me to see them as an audit trail and helped me to write a short essay that I added at the end, which I called 'journeying'. I got the student prize for insights associated with that work – the way I dealt with uncertainty within my studies.

Activity 10.2   *Critical thinking*

Prepare a single paragraph of writing that you think demonstrates critical thinking, which attends to a stated learning outcome and shows that you are approaching care with due concern for the context or clientele of your practice. To help others evaluate your paragraph, state the learning outcome above your short piece of work. We have included an excerpt from one of Fatima's portfolio entries at the end of this chapter for you to compare with your own. What do your work and hers have in common? If one entry seems better than the other, why is this?

Next, repeat the process, preparing a short plan for future learning, either one drawn from your own portfolio, or one that seems important to you now and you draft from scratch. Refer to Table 10.1 above as an aide-memoire of what should feature in your plan. What lessons do you draw from a review of your own and Fatima's offering?

As stated, the extract from Fatima's portfolio can be found at the end of the chapter.

Reflection and your portfolio

We discussed the process of reflective writing at some length in Chapter 9, so here we propose sharing with you some more specific thoughts on reflective writing that draw together the individual reflections that you have developed earlier. We call this process 'synthesis of learning' and it can, at best, demonstrate your ability to theorise about nursing care. A simple analogy can help us to demonstrate the value of this. Imagine that you are staring up into the night sky and you spot a particularly bright star. You study this using some binoculars. You learn something about that star, its colour and magnitude of light perhaps. But to make better sense of stars, and our position in relation to stars and galaxies, we need to gather together a collection of such observations. We need to spot the position of stars in the sky and to note that stars seem to be clustered more densely in one part of the sky than another. In this way, we learn something about galaxies and, with some extra reading, discover something about our own galaxy and our position within it. The area of dense stars is where we look into the Milky Way and understand our position towards the edge of that galaxy. Linking reflections together can be like the comparison of stars and the realisation that they seem to form some sort of pattern. If we start to recognise patterns, perhaps some that recur again and again, we start to theorise what is happening. We begin to anticipate what we might see next and to speculate about why this happens.

For such an overarching reflection to work it needs to involve a series of steps.

- Identifying all the relevant experiences and indicating why these constitute a group (Fatima started these entries by listing all the preceding references that were being discussed and stating in a line or two what they were all about. In one instance, this was 'effective listening').
- Comparing and contrasting experiences. This means showing experiences that seem to signal the same thing and others that remind us that neat explanations might not be possible. With regard to effective listening, for instance, Fatima noted that experiences repeatedly emphasised the importance of adequate time, privacy and attention, if listening was to be effective. She noted, however, that patients varied in their need for feedback on what had been understood by the nurse. Some needed the nurse to summarise what had been understood, while others were content that the nurse had simply given of her time.
- Speculating what this tells us. As with individual reflections, we need to determine what (if anything) the experiences tell us. It is necessary at this level, where several reflections are brought together, to be especially cautious about overstating what the experience means. We need to identify the limits of what experience seems to explain, and to note where any resultant, working theory starts to falter. Fatima determined that, while we might ideally wish to provide patients with a summary of what is gleaned from their account of problems or needs, it seemed sometimes sufficient to report back just the highlights. This would be enough to reassure a large number of patients of our appreciation of their needs. There were, however, exceptions to this principle, especially where patients were talking about matters relating to informed consent. There, and in other areas where patient safety was important, it was critical to indicate exactly all that had been understood.
- Determining what follows next. While actions may be possible with reference to individual reflections (e.g., I won't assume that all patients have enough funds to easily secure a balanced diet), further enquiries and discussions may be the more common outcome for reflections that draw on several experiences. This was important in Fatima's example, because the reputation of nurses, as advocates, as carers and as communicators, rested upon how effective listening was understood and used. In her portfolio entry, therefore, she reported that she took the observations to a clinical update meeting for the ward nurses and that it provoked a thoughtful debate. Registered nurse colleagues complimented her on her analysis and started to reflect on their own experiences afresh.

Critical thinking

Consider now whether, as a result of several learning experiences, those in clinical settings and beyond, you are starting to formulate working theories, tentative explanations of how nursing works, and what is important in the delivery of nursing care. At best, these are likely to relate to the support of a given patient group, or perhaps to techniques or processes that are used again and again by nurses (e.g., patient education, discharge planning, referral to social service agencies). The focus of your interest should be relatively discrete, as Fatima's was. Follow the above steps to formulate a tentative working theory about these matters that you can share with study group colleagues and your tutor. Your written entry to the portfolio at this stage will be in rough form. It is open to modification as a result of the conversations that you next share with colleagues. There will be opportunity during the study group conversation for you to defend your points, to consider alternative observations and to connect these discoveries to some of the theory that you may have been taught.

As this activity is based on your own reflection, there is no answer at the end of the chapter.

While we can only guess what you deliberate on and what you then conclude, our experience suggests that even quite modest series of experiences can start to generate reflections that might support a very tentative theory on one aspect of practice. Students we have supported have shared reflections on aspects of patient care, on implementing healthcare policy, on the nature of practice innovation and on multi-disciplinary working, to name but a few. The subsequent group discussions have then served to modify or augment the theory and to suggest a new round of observations or enquiries that might enable the nurse to test these ideas further. While this reflective entry appears in section 2 of the portfolio, it has often generated a new entry in section 3. Fatima, too, generated a new action plan in association with her reflections on active listening and began to ask patients what they most valued when nurses fed back on the conversations shared with them. She started to search for the recurring, patient-valued elements of feedback by nurses, so that these could be used more frequently in her own practice.

Sharing group discussions about a working theory enables you to join together reflection and critical thinking. You have begun to formulate ideas about care as a result of several reflections, and now the support/challenge/questions that you encounter in group discussion enable you to deepen your analysis. This is frequently how nursing care is refined and improved. One colleague shares an observation with several others and comparisons are made regarding what has been discovered. Each then explores what remains to be understood, what might enhance care and what could be done to improve the knowledge or skill of the practitioner. While research can certainly fuel practice improvements, critically discussed reflections can too. Your portfolio becomes the record of that process.

Making the case regarding your development

While your portfolio may well be submitted for assessment purposes at one or more points within your course, there is a sense in which it never quite ends as a product. There is always something more that could be added, or something that could be modified in the light of a new enquiry or experience. Using your portfolio, though, taking it beyond personal reflection, is vital. If you never share your reflections and claims with others, there is every possibility that you might delude yourself regarding what is important, effective, professional or needful in nursing. There are a number of junctures, therefore, where you share the portfolio with others and use it to make the case regarding your professional development, for example:

- sharing end of module or annual work with your personal tutor (this tutor is interested in the different themes of your development and may make recommendations with regard to these);
- showing work to colleagues at the end of a clinical placement (sometimes mentors are asked to review clinical placement reflections from the portfolio with you);
- submitting the work for gateway assessment (portfolio-based learning is frequently used in nursing and you may need to satisfy portfolio requirements to proceed to the next stage or level of your course);
- demonstrating to others that you have successfully completed a probationary period of practice after registration as a nurse, or on moving into a specialist field of work;
- demonstrating to an employer or other authority that your learning is up to date and that you remain fit to practise, at either a standard or a more advanced practice level.

Requirements vary regarding what within the portfolio you are required to show. As we noted above, the NMC requirements focus especially on reflective records of different kinds, which might typically be drawn from section 2 of the portfolio. For annual appraisal purposes, the post-registration review of your work, or for module assessment purposes, other select elements of the portfolio might need to be submitted and discussed. You may, for example, need to submit records of placement learning out-comes successfully met (with mentor signatures) and a series of reflections that capture your discoveries there. In most instances, personal tutors like to see an overview of your development, but for many others it is an excerpt of the portfolio that you will submit.

It can feel strange, even unsettling, to share elements of your work after what may have seemed very private reflection. Portfolios of learning, however, remain at least semi-public documents, open to review by examiners and, sometimes, those charged with investigating malpractice. Even if you are not under investigation yourself, you may still hold a record that sheds light on incidents involving another practitioner. We suggest, therefore, that you write the portfolio always as though entries could be inspected by others. It is important to date entries and link them to the places where the experiences were shared. Later, where the law or codes of conduct requirements dictate, you may be asked to elaborate on your entries.

A well-structured and organised portfolio will already make significant points about your professionalism. It demonstrates your critical thought and reflection. But to use the portfolio to best effect, with a current purpose in mind, you must have read it recently and considered how it addresses the requirements of the day. For example, what within the portfolio points to your abilities as required in a job description? What is it about your portfolio that shows your commitment and interest in a particular field of practice that you hope to move into? Taking the time to reread your portfolio and to draw key points from it that you might add to a letter of application, use in an interview or include within a presentation will enhance your chances of success. The same point holds good in 'open book' examinations, where students are allowed to bring notes, including excerpts from their portfolios, into the examination room. What are the most relevant entries here? There won't be time to find and refer to everything in such settings, so identify what is most pertinent to the requirements of the day.

Activity 10.4   *Critical thinking*

Return to Activity 10.1 and consider whether you should now add to your list of bullet points describing the advantages of building a portfolio.

- Had you previously considered how the portfolio can demonstrate your style of reasoning, and your attitudes and approach to others? This might be advantageous if your attitudes were subsequently questioned.
- Does it serve to show your inquisitiveness and commitment to learning, something that might be reviewed if you struggled with a certain section of your course or if a special award was being considered?
- Does your portfolio become an important resource when you seek a post in a much-favoured clinical area of practice – could this provide the edge that helps you to secure the post?

Update your bullet point list now and refer to it periodically if your interest in portfolio building and maintenance starts to flag.

As this activity is based on your own reflection, there is no answer at the end of the chapter.

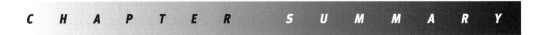

C   H   A   P   T   E   R   S   U   M   M   A   R   Y

In this chapter, we have considered what a portfolio consists of and how it relates to the critical thinking and reflection that are so much a part of nursing courses and professional practice. We have made the case that, while building and maintaining a portfolio can seem onerous (especially if you are not naturally inclined towards making diary entries), there are distinct advantages, as well as professional responsibilities, associated with portfolio work. The portfolio has a utilitarian purpose – it can be used as evidence of your achievements, abilities and potential. It becomes a vehicle for enhanced thinking and working, as you start to examine how and why care could or should be different. At best, it fuels the process of theorising – something that nurses should engage in wherever they are worried about practice. Writing up reflections that synthesise a series of experiences and past reflections made at the time can help you to think more conceptually and 'out of the box' (i.e., more creatively).

At its very best, building and using a portfolio is not something that you arrange secretively. It becomes part of the fabric of collective learning. You get into the habit of comparing notes with colleagues, reflections, excerpts from what you have read and examples of research evidence that you wish to evaluate and perhaps use. The portfolio is, therefore, a vehicle for professional discourse, which enables us to sustain our interest in nursing and the enrichment of nursing care.

All of the above, however, starts with much more prosaic first steps. You need to arrange the portfolio in a clear, accessible and consistent manner. You need to set up sections and entries in such a way that you can cross-reference material; only then does it enable you to show how you combine insights to demonstrate your understanding. You need to select what goes into the portfolio, accept that some first entries may be tentative or rough, and remain open to adjustment or refinement. Arranging the portfolio in loose-leaf or computer-based form provides that kind of flexibility. You can add to the portfolio and take away from it, at will.

In the craft guilds of the Middle Ages, one of the first things that an apprentice did was to build or design a tool that they used during the rest of their career. Their first work was to create a model – a template that guided some of their practice as a master craftsperson. In many regards, portfolio building does exactly this. You build a tool for your use that can serve you well for a very long time. It is worth the investment.

Activities: brief outline answers and reflections

Activity 10.2: Critical thinking (page 134)

Extract from Fatima's critical thinking work

Learning outcome: The student will be able to, in association with the patient and other relevant stakeholders, develop a nursing care plan that reflects relevant priorities and needs.

During my placement on Ivy ward I engaged in three episodes of care planning, each with a different patient and experienced nurse in attendance. As this is a surgical ward, with a large number of patients staying with us for relatively short periods of time (2–4 days), and as there are standard protocols for the majority of care delivered, my individualised care planning centred either on what supplemented the standard protocol, or on variations to the protocol mandated by the patient's circumstances. Care planning had to demonstrate due regard for the patient as an individual, determine what was realisable during the hospital stay (other care might be recommended post-discharge) and work with the available resources (other patients competed for our attention, so we needed to plan for the needs of the group as well as the needs of the individual). I noted that, while all the registered nurses recommended slightly different approaches to collaboration in care planning, all were referenced against what I describe as 'practice consequences'. One registered nurse said to me, 'Imagine what would happen if you did do this and what might happen if you didn't. You need to weigh up the benefits and the costs of care, especially if you agree a plan that you expect others to contribute to.' I practised with that idea in mind then, and discovered that all three patients appreciated my efforts to personalise care as far as possible. They hadn't expected 'tailor-made care', were well aware of the pressures on hospital beds, but applauded my extra questions: about what the patients did normally, what they found easiest or most worthwhile and what frightened or encouraged them.

Our notes

We suggest that this ably shows Fatima addressing the learning outcome, as she demonstrates a due regard for patients and acknowledges their part in care planning. In addition, though, there is a clear recognition here of the constraints upon joint care planning. Resources are finite and the plans cannot be unlimited. The stakeholders acknowledged here, then, are the patient, other patients on the ward and the healthcare professionals who must balance the priorities of care. A further benefit of this passage is that she indicates how the learning is achieved – through discussion and observation with three different nurses. This shows how Fatima is able to synthesise information from different sources.

Now, here is the example of an outline plan that Fatima prepared for another element of her learning. Fatima was interested in identifying how nurses on Ivy ward evaluated their daily care-giving efforts. She believed that feeling good about the shift completed was important if a career was to be sustained in nursing. Several of the nurses seemed hard-pressed in their work, but also very content with what they achieved.

Aim

To identify what, within care giving in a ward shift, sustains registered nurses in their commitment to nursing work, that is, what gives them personal satisfaction.

Method

1. Observations of selected nurses who share the same shifts as me.
2. Brief discussions with each of them, about what sustains them and helps them to always try to improve their contribution.

Support

The nurses themselves are my chief resource, but I will also look in the library for a textbook on the psychology of work. While that book might not be on nursing, I think it might have something to offer anyway.

Time-frame

I will continue with this work for the remainder of my clinical placement, which is just over a month, ending in March 2010.

Achievement proof

I will be able to list three or four key things that help sustain a nurse in their work. To each item on that list I will then add a reflection on the extent to which I have developed same.

Our notes

We were impressed with the clarity and the precision of this plan. It is opportunistic – learning will happen as and when Fatima can observe and speak with the nurses concerned, but the approach is coherent and impressively supported by the idea of dipping into a book on the psychology of work. While it is an unconventional action plan, focusing on the meaning of nursing work rather than clinical skills, we thought it a very valid one. What sustains a career is interest in what we achieve on a daily basis. We admired the way that Fatima has also anticipated what would constitute achievement in this work, which is important given that this is not something routinely assessed by the college.

Knowledge review

In order to check your grasp of the above material, address the following questions, returning to Chapter 10 where you struggle to provide an answer.

1. Name five advantages in building and using a portfolio in nursing.
2. How will you arrange the layout of your own portfolio, and what is the rationale for the sections that you use?

3. What is it about portfolio building and use that enables you to demonstrate your critical thinking?
4. What is involved in writing a reflection of a series of past episodes and why is this important for nurses?
5. You are about to go for an interview, write an examination paper or meet up with your personal tutor to discuss progress. What should you do now to ensure that your portfolio serves you well in these situations?

Further reading

Hopson, B and Ledger, K (2009) *And What Do You Do? 10 steps to creating a portfolio career*. London: A & C Black.
It may surprise you that one of our recommended reads concerns not your portfolio during student years, but the use of a portfolio afterwards! Straightforward, linear careers are not so common in nursing any more, and colleagues frequently shift their field of work, their geographical location or their roles, as well as decide whether to work full or part time. Thus, developing a portfolio that accommodates changing aspirations and circumstances is important, and this accessible book tells you all about how to do that.

Pearce, R (2006) *Foundations in Nursing and Healthcare: Profiles and portfolios of evidence*. Cheltenham: Nelson Thornes.
Our second recommendation comes from more familiar territory and offers you a whole text solely on portfolio building. The work is accessible and practical, and comes with a CD-ROM that offers different templates for your own portfolio (a key selling point).

Useful websites

www.ecu.edu.au/CLT/pdf/tl_portfolio.pdf
Bunker, A (2005) *The Teaching and Learning Portfolio at ECU: Demonstrating scholarship in teaching and learning*. Prepared for Learning Resources Development, Edith Cowan University, Western Australia.
We have been struck by how much is written for students about profiling, portfolio development and learning logs, and how little there is for tutors who often lead such approaches to learning. This, then, is a modest but accessible pdf document that rebalances matters. Bunker highlights how different sorts of evidence and discussion within a teacher's own portfolio can demonstrate his or her education and management skills.

www.journalofnursingeducation.com/ShowFree.asp?thing=3472
Kear, M and Bear, M (2007) Using portfolio evaluation for program outcome assessment. *Journal of Nursing Education*, 46(3): 109–14.
Go to the above web address and click on the 'back issues' button on the left. Type 'kear' into the search box to bring up a PDF of this article by two American nurse authors on the business of assessing portfolios within nurse education. Nursing students are proving increasingly adept, skilful and confident in the building of learning portfolios, so it is important to use assessment systems that match developments. Excellent work in portfolio building deserves the award of high marks, but we must be clear about how such marks were achieved! While this paper reports a relatively modest and interim piece of research, many of the reflections shared here are relevant to our work with portfolios and the assessment of learning.

References

Ashby, C (2006) Models for reflective practice. *Practice Nurse,* 32(10): 28–32.

Baxter Magolda, M (1992) *Knowing and Reasoning in College Students: Gender-related patterns in students' intellectual development.* San Francisco, CA: Jossey-Bass.

Belenky, M, Clinchy, B, Goldberger, R and Tarule, J (1986) *Women's Ways of Knowing.* New York: Basic Books.

Brooker, C and Waugh, W (2007) *Foundation of Nursing Practice: Fundamentals of holistic care.* St Louis, MO: Mosby.

Bulman, C and Schutz S (2008) *Reflective Practice in Nursing,* 4th edition. Oxford: Blackwell.

Burnard, P and Gill, P (2008) *Culture, Communication and Nursing: A multicultural guide.* Harlow: Pearson Education.

Carper, B (2004) Fundamental patterns of knowing, in Reed, P, Shearer, N and Nicoll, L (eds) *Perspectives in Nursing Theory,* Philadelphia, PA: Lippincott, Williams and Wilkins, pp221–8.

Carroll, R (2009) *Risk Management Handbook for Health Care Organizations (student edition).* San Francisco, CA: Jossey-Bass.

Cortazzi, M and Jin, L (1997) Communicating for learning across cultures, in McNamara, D and Harris, R (eds) *Overseas Students in Higher Education: Issues in teaching and learning.* London: Routledge, pp76–90.

Craig, C (2009) Learning about reflections through exploring narrative enquiry. *Reflective Practice,* 10(1): 105–16.

de Bono, E (2000) *Six Thinking Hats: Run better meetings, make faster decisions.* London: Penguin.

Dunlosky, J and Metcalfe, J (2008) *Metacognition: A textbook for cognitive, educational, lifespan and applied psychology.* Thousand Oaks, CA: Sage.

Gibbs, G (1988) *Learning By Doing: A guide to teaching and learning methods.* Oxford: Oxford Polytechnic Further Education Unit.

Gobet, F (2005) Chunking models of expertise: implications for education. *Applied Cognitive Psychology,* 19: 183–204.

Hek, G, Singer, L and Taylor, P (2004) Cross-boundary working: a generic worker for older people in the community. *British Journal of Community Nursing,* 9(6): 237–44.

Howatson-Jones, L (2010) *Reflective Practice in Nursing.* Exeter: Learning Matters.

Jasper, M (2003) *Foundations in Nursing and Health Care: Beginning reflective practice.* London: Nelson Thornes.

Joel, L (2009) *Advanced Practice in Nursing: Essentials for role development,* 2nd edition. Philadelphia, PA: FA Davis.

Johns, C (1995) Framing learning through reflection within Carper's fundamental ways of knowing in nursing. *Journal of Advanced Nursing,* 22: 226–34.

Kassirer, J, Wong, J and Kopelman, R (2009) *Learning Clinical Reasoning,* 2nd edition. Philadelphia, PA: Lippincott, Williams and Wilkins.

Kinnell, D and Hughes, P (2010) *Mentoring Nursing and Healthcare Students.* Thousand Oaks, CA: Sage.

Kirpal, S (2004) Work identities of nurses: between caring and efficiency demands. *Career Development International,* 9(3): 274–304.

Leuf, B and Cunningham, W (2002) *What Is Wiki?* Available online at http://wiki.org/wiki.cgi?WhatIsWiki (accessed 15 January 2010).

Lucas, R (2009) *Training Workshop Essentials: Designing, developing and delivering learning events that get results.* San Francisco, CA: Pfeiffer.

Mardell, J and Serfozo, K (2010) *Personal Injury and Clinical Negligence Litigation.* Guildford: College of Law Publishing.

Marsick, V and O'Neil, J (2007) *Understanding Action Learning: Theory into practice.* New York: Amacon.

McCance, T, Slater, P and McCormack, B (2009) Using the caring dimensions inventory as an indicator of person-centred nursing. *Journal of Clinical Nursing,* 18: 409–17.

McCray, J (2009) *Nursing and Multiprofessional Practice.* Thousand Oaks, CA: Sage.

McDonald, S, Henderson, J, Faulkner, S, Evans, S and Hagan, R (2010) Effect of an extended midwifery postnatal support programme on the duration of breastfeeding: a randomized control trial. *Midwifery,* 26(1): 88–100.

McGrath, P (1990) *Pain in Children: Nature, assessment and treatment.* New York: Guilford Press.

Moody, H (2004) Hospital discharge planning: carrying out orders? *Journal of Gerontological Social Work,* 43(1): 107–18.

Moon, J (2008) *Critical Thinking: An exploration of theory and practice.* London: Routledge.

Nursing and Midwifery Council (NMC) (2008) *The Code: Standards of conduct, performance and ethics for nurses and midwives.* London: NMC.

Nursing and Midwifery Council (NMC) (2010a) *The Prep Handbook.* London: NMC. Available online at www.nmc-uk.org/aDisplayDocument.aspx?documentID=4340 (accessed 24 March 2010).

Nursing and Midwifery Council (NMC) (2010b) *Standards for pre-registration nursing education.* London: NMC.

Pearson, A (2003) Multidisciplinary nursing: rethinking role boundaries. *Journal of Clinical Nursing,* 12(5): 625–9.

Pearson, A, Field, J and Jordan, Z (2007) *Evidence-based Clinical Practice in Nursing and Healthcare: A comprehensive approach to evidence-based practice in nursing and the health professions.* Oxford: Blackwell.

Price, B (2003a) *Studying Nursing using Problem-based and Enquiry-based Learning.* Basingstoke: Palgrave.

Price, B (2003b) Academic voices and the challenges of tutoring. *Nurse Education Today,* 23(8): 628–37.

Price, B (2005) Thinking aloud your practice. *Nursing Standard,* 19(31): supplement.

Race, P (2007) *The Lecturer's Toolkit: A practical guide to assessment, learning and teaching.* Abingdon: Routledge.

Schon, D (1987) *Educating the Reflective Practitioner.* San Francisco, CA: Jossey-Bass.

Seedhouse, D (2000) *Practical Nursing Philosophy: The universal ethical code.* Chichester: Wiley.

Seedhouse, D (2009) *Ethics: The heart of healthcare,* 3rd edition. Chichester: Wiley.

Slote, M (2007) *The Ethics of Care and Empathy.* Abingdon: Routledge.

Speck, P (2006) *Teamwork in Palliative Care: Fulfilling or frustrating?* Oxford: Oxford University Press.

Stuart, C (2007) *Assessment, Supervision and Support in Clinical Practice: A guide for nurses, midwives and other health professionals*, 2nd edition. Edinburgh: Churchill Livingstone.

Thompson, C and Dowding, D (2009) *Essential Decision Making and Clinical Judgement for Nurses*. Edinburgh: Churchill Livingstone.

Wicks, E (2007) *Human Rights and Healthcare*. Portland, OR: Hart Publishing.

Index